NATALIE

NATALIE
Barry and Cathy Beaver

as told to
Darryl E. Hicks

HUNTINGTON HOUSE INC.

Shreveport • Lafayette
Louisiana

Copyright ©1985 by Barry and Cathy Beaver
ISBN Number 0-910311-27-7
Printed in the United States of America
Library of Congress Catalog Card Number: 85-60776

All rights reserved. No part of this book may be reproduced without permission from the publisher, except by a reviewer who may quote brief passages in a review; nor may any part of this book be reproduced, stored in a retrieval system or copied by mechanical, photocopying, recording or other means, without permission from the publisher.

Photographs by Pam Hardister and Bob Grundisch

ACKNOWLEDGEMENTS

To our parents — Thurman and Phyllis Wood, J.C. and Edith Beaver, and to all our family who encouraged us, supported us, and prayed with us as we lived these pages.

To the hospital staff at the pediatric intensive care unit, Charlotte Memorial Hospital, for their love and care for all the children and for us.

All Scripture references from the King James Version, unless otherwise noted.

"My Tribute" (pages 13, 14, 15, 16 and 136), by Andrae Crouch, Copyright © 1971 by Lexicon Music, Inc. Used by permission.

"We've Come This Far by Faith" (page 132), by Albert Goodson, Copyright © 1963 by Manna Music, Inc., 2111 Kenmere Ave., Burbank, CA 91504. International copyright service. All rights reserved. Used by permission.

DEDICATION

To the Lord — who put all the pieces together, from beginning to end.

> *God is not a man, that He should tell or act a lie, neither the son of man, that He should feel repentance or compunction (for what He has promised). Has He said, and shall He not do it? Or has He spoken and shall He not make it good? (Numbers 23:19, Amplified Bible)*

FOREWORD

When I first met Natalie Beaver several years ago, I was moved — of course — by her incredible, "impossible" story.

So when I received this book, I relived that initial shock, disbelief, hurt, and dread. But I also felt emerging faith as I saw Barry and Cathy's gritty, never-say-die courage.

Natalie is a frank, thoughtful, and self-revealing look at both a horrible tragedy *and* the people who simply refused to let go.

The agonies and victories are etched page after page. I know many lives will be changed after being touched by little Natalie. Many already have.

Pat Boone

TABLE OF CONTENTS

		Page
1	Tribute	13
2	Promise For A Dark Night	17
3	It Wasn't Connected!	21
4	Flashing Lights	28
5	Pain, Pressure, And A Little Faith	31
6	Alone Together	43
7	No End In Sight	48
8	Not By Sight	54
9	Empty Bed	76
10	Cruel Tape... Shaking Hands	113
11	This Far By Faith	125
12	Sharing The Light	133

1

TRIBUTE

*How can I say thanks
  for the things You have done for me?
Things so undeserved,
  yet You give to prove Your love for me.
The voices of a million angels
  could not express my gratitude;
All that I am and ever hope to be —
  I owe it all to Thee.*

We stand, like so many others, in the wings of the television studio as enthralled as the national audience. Our little Natalie is singing her heart out.

Neither of us — even as parents — have quite gotten over how naturally she sings. It seems to flow effortlessly. Even her expressions are innate. Special.

All parents think their own children are extremely special, like us. Funny thing though — others have always been more amazed with her talent than us.

We see our daughter every day, in playclothes romping out in the backyard with our dog; with chocolate cookie smeared across her impish grin. We put her to bed at night and watch her cuddle up with her favorite doll. She's our daughter. It would be very easy, since we are up close every day, to glance past how especially anointed she is. Other people remind us though. And we know it most keenly when she sings.

> *To God be the glory,*
> *To God be the glory,*
> *To God be the glory,*
>   *For the things He has done*

By the time she was four, she was already singing in front of people. No stage parents — we! In fact, we couldn't keep her away from the platform once she tasted the response her little voice could bring.

But that was several years ago. Some pretty big doors have opened since then. Churches. Schools. Charity telethons. Local broadcasts. Regional stations. Satellite network programs reaching into the nation's homes.

Tribute

It's all been pretty heady stuff for a small girl like Natalie.

> *With His blood He has saved me,*
> *With His pow'r He has raised me,*
> *To God be the glory for the things*
>   *He has done.*

People are surprised when they hear our little girl sing. Back home in North Carolina, we call it "beltin' out a song." She does that with her eyes a-sparkling!

But the most amazing part is not Natalie's singing. It's her story.

When we begin sharing her beginning, there are varied responses, of course, especially when we show pictures of her at birth.

Some people are repulsed, sure. Most are mainly shocked. Intrigued. We've seen most moved to tears at the thought of such a thing.

> *Just let me live my life —*
>   *Let it be pleasing Lord to Thee;*
> *And should I gain any praise*
>   *Let it go to Calvary.*

Natalie was born premature with most of her internal organs on the outside of her tiny body. Her chances of living were one in millions. The doctors made it clear, from the beginning, that she would not, could not survive.

They kept on saying that even when she did.

With His blood He has saved me,
With His pow'r He has raised me,
To God be the glory for the things
   He has done.

Many have already been touched by Natalie's story, but what they haven't understood is the struggle behind the dramatic chain of events. The hurts. The absolute depressions. The lessons. God's miraculous power.

Maybe it's time everything was told — the good, the gruesome, and the darkest moments when the shadows could have easily overpowered the flickering light.

These things — not just the beautiful little brown-haired girl all dressed up in the shiny blue dress, not just the small songbird bringing lumps to the throats of so many across the states — these things make up Natalie's *real* story.

2

PROMISE FOR A DARK NIGHT

Sunday, November 9, 1975.

CATHY:

I had already been through a nightmarish pregnancy. Nauseous. They didn't even know that I was pregnant for four months since I had a backwards uterus. I knew something wasn't right.

But it was reaching a crescendo. I was getting sicker by the day. I had been through false labors and rush trips to the hospital already.

It happened again. Barry and I went through another hurried, harried trip to the hospital. Again, nothing. More pain. That was all.

But that night my brother, Jeff Wood, and his wife came by. He mentioned the service he'd preached in the nearby church where he pastored — "God really moved. There were special miracles taking place..."

But I was in pain. I didn't want to hear about all the other things.

"Jeff," I cried, "I am really sick!" That's all I said. I made my point.

My brother came around to the other side of the bed. Almost instantly he began speaking a prophetic word that we all realized was from God — "I'll protect you and that which is within you, because I am your God, and I will restore you to perfect health!"

The words were powerful. They hit us like lightning bolts. Little did I know just how special they would be during the coming days and nights.

In fact, those words became the key, the basis of everything. EVERYTHING.

Wednesday, November 19, 1975.

CATHY:

My mother was right beside me in my maternity room at the Cabarrus Hospital in Concord, North Carolina.

I started hurting bad about 2 a.m. At 2:30 or so I finally grabbed mother's arm and squeezed it as hard as I could.

"Mother, I can't take anymore!"

Then I looked up. "God, I can't take anymore!"

My eyes met mother's — "You better get a nurse in here right now!"

She did. The nurse started screaming because she saw that the baby was already coming out.

Another nurse ran in — "Mrs. Beaver, you've got to hold your labor because the doctor isn't here yet."

Well, that was like asking me to hold back Niagara Falls. I was much too far gone for that.

The next thing I remember was the doctor talking to me. I couldn't wake up. He was telling me things about my baby which I couldn't understand. Everything went black again.

Then I remember my daddy talking to me. He was also telling me about the baby.

I still didn't understand.

BARRY:

Another false alarm. I had rushed Cathy to the hospital again in yet another futile attempt during an ever-increasingly strange pregnancy.

By 10 that night, at everyone's insistence, I left Cathy's room and went home to get a few hours sleep. I was scheduled to sing on four television tapings the next day. Wakeup was coming early for me to get ready.

I was sound asleep at 1:30 a.m. when the phone shattered the silence in my room. It was Thurman Wood, Cathy's father.

"Barry, they're taking Cathy into the delivery room. This time it's the real thing!"

We had been through this several times, so I took my time showering and getting dressed. I was still thinking about the television taping, figuring that I might not have time to get home and get dressed for that if I had to stay at the hospital for a while.

Thurman met me when I steered my car under the floodlights of the hospital parking lot. That made me realize how urgent the situation was.

I jumped from the car and ran up to the floor where I had left my wife just a few hours before.

I was too late to see her. She had already gone into labor by then. The traditional "wait" began.

But none of us knew how untraditional the result would be. None of us knew either that the dark night was just beginning. It would be a long, nightmarish time before the dawn.

3

IT WASN'T CONNECTED!!

BARRY:

I arrived at the hospital sometime around 2:30 a.m. I was already thinking about all that Cathy had gone through during the pregnancy. The entire time — almost eight months — had been marked by horrible nausea. As the birth neared, two weeks before, when the contractions and false labor pains began, she had vomited so much that she became dehydrated.

She had grown so large (in size) that when the doctors did the amniocentesis, where fluid is removed from the womb to be tested, I remembered Dr. Monroe just letting a lot of fluid run through. He had said, "There's so much in there, that some needs to be let out." The Lord really had his hand even in this — if the baby had gone full term, and if so much fluid had remained in there, the liquid would have backed up into Cathy's lungs. She would have literally drowned, and the baby would have obviously gone too.

But God had given the prophecy to Cathy — "I'll protect you and that which is within you, because I am your God, and I will restore you to perfect health!"

I wasn't thinking about those words as I sat waiting in the hospital lounge. As the clock neared three that morning, the activity hit a flurry.

At this point we knew that there were two or three other ladies in the delivery area and that all their babies had already been delivered. We knew that Cathy was the only one left back there.

By this time, I was getting real worried. It was ironic — I wasn't really thinking about the baby. I was worried about Cathy. A nurse and orderly came running out of the room. Within seconds, they ran back in with oxygen tanks. I remember Cathy's daddy getting up then; he was almost white as a sheet — his wife (Phyllis) went through a real bad time with Jeff, their son — so he was obviously reliving that.

When I looked at him, I really came apart. I was looking for something to hold onto. He

It Wasn't Connected!!

looked like he was coming apart, so there seemed to be nothing left. I didn't even think to call on God at that point. My mind was scrambled eggs. I didn't understand what was going on. I thought, "Here I am, 27 years old, and I've never had a real crisis to deal with in my life. If Cathy dies, I don't think I can handle it."

Anyway, they ran in with the oxygen tanks. It was a waiting game for us. The waiting room, however, was empty for everyone except Thurman, Phyllis and myself.

They told us later that it was 3:02 a.m. when our baby was born. I guess that was right. We didn't know. All we saw was a lot of anxiety on everyone's face as each hurried in and out. I could tell that something wasn't right. The nurses wouldn't look into our faces. It was like they didn't want to say anything — I'm sure that they had been told not to say anything.

"Is there anything wrong?" I asked.

One nurse admitted, "Well, we don't know." Wow! That plunged us further into panic.

I had talked about all this "faith in God" stuff and how people can overcome. Here I was, hit by an obstacle that I had never known, and I didn't know how to overcome it at all. I had been genuine in my words before — but it seemed like my blocks had been knocked out from under me. I didn't have anything to hold onto. Everything was blown apart by the shock and panic. I felt so helpless, not knowing if Cathy was alive or dead. Again, I wasn't even thinking about the baby. I was just thinking of all the horrible things that could be happening to Cathy.

Then they came out pushing the isolette with my baby in it. The doctor walked in front, hurriedly — "There's something wrong, Mr. Beaver." My heart was pumping wildly.

At that point I felt like a spectator — like I was just listening in on someone else's conversation. There were two nurses standing there with Dr. Monroe. They had our baby lying in the isolette. I could see the lights reflected on the glassy, bubble-like covering. The baby had blue sterile towels over her midsection, but I saw her face. She was crying like all babies are supposed to. I couldn't understand why the doctor was telling me that there was something wrong with the baby. Phyllis and Thurman were standing on the side. I started to ask what was wrong but before I could, Dr. Monroe reached inside the openings on the side of the isolette, pushed his hands through the sterile gloves and pulled the towels back.

From that point on, I didn't hear too much of what he said. I was totally in shock.

Time has not diminished that incredibly vivid sight imprinted in my memory of that moment.

I could see this hopeless looking mass of insides. It was a living anatomy class — just like in college. I saw her liver, bladder, gall bladder, spleen, stomach, intestines — everything!

I'd seen pictures in college biology classes. I'd even seen the details on human fetuses. But that was different. This baby was still alive.

I could see the blood running through the vessels and veins. I kept staring at that throbbing mass of stomach, and yet I could look up at my baby's little face — it was perfectly normal. She had such distinct features — her eyebrows, eyes and mouth, black hair. I could see that she was very much alive. And yet — the stomach. That pitiful, completely abnormal mass.

I looked at Dr. Monroe. Phyllis was frantic. Crying. It was just too much for her to handle. Thurman was trying to hold her up. I don't think I was crying at that point. I must have been glassy-eyed. I didn't have the foggiest idea of what was going on. Dr. Monroe was talking — something about the fact that they had already called the ambulance service to get up there. They were going to send the baby to Charlotte Memorial Hospital.

Like a slow-motion sequence from a grade-B movie, the events continued with me just reacting, not really understanding what was happening.

I watched as Dr. Monroe reached inside the isolette again, covered the baby girl up, and let the orderlies push the contraption down the hall to wait for the ambulance attendants.

Dr. Monroe walked a few steps away. I was alone there. Thurman was trying to take care of Phyllis in the waiting room.

I looked at the doctor's sweat-soaked togs. He was shaking his head and mumbling — "It wasn't connected."

I was grabbing for straws, not able to understand what he was saying. By then I was starting to react to the entire situation. It was beginning to dawn on me that the baby's stomach-thing had been going on all during the pregnancy. The medical people hadn't known. "What kind of doctors do we have?" I thought. "How could they not know what was going on inside?"

At that point, I didn't know anything about the gravity of the problem. I was, as mentioned before, grabbing for straws. It infuriated me that the doctor kept mumbling something about not being connected.

I said, "What do you mean, it wasn't connected? What are you talking about?"

I looked at him. My eyes were crackling fire. My little baby was 30 feet down the hall by then. I had no idea whether she would live or die. And he was mumbling something that made no sense.

"What wasn't connected?" I demanded.

He said, "The umbilical cord."

"You mean it broke off when she was born?"

"No," he breathed wearily, "it just wasn't connected to anything. It was *never* connected

It Wasn't Connected!! 27

to anything!"

I was growing more irritated by the moment— "I still don't understand — 'not connected to anything.' That's the life line! I took biology. That's the only way the baby could have received any nourishment. That's the only way the baby could have lived inside the womb!"

He shook his head again, his deep-set eyes seemed focused on something far away. "It wasn't connected. It was formed from conception that way."

I couldn't help being skeptical. "If she was like this from the beginning, how did she grow?"

But he didn't answer me. He didn't know. I asked him several more times, but he didn't have any answers.

Not connected! How could it be? The entire scene was growing more nightmarish with each passing moment.

4

FLASHING LIGHTS

BARRY:

The first thoughts, as I stood alone once again in the hallway, were — "Lord, if she's gonna have trouble, I'd just as soon you'd take her home. She'd be better off."

I got so convicted, instantly, in my heart that I would even think such a thought. I recognized it was the evil one who had planted it.

Maybe that was the first point where I started to reach down and feel a little spark of faith. I kicked the Satan-inspired thought out of my head — "I'm not going to believe that!"

Just then the ambulance drivers arrived and the attendants summoned me to go with them.

Flashing Lights

They said that they had to have a parent there in Charlotte when they arrived to give vital admissions information.

Mr. and Mrs. Wood stayed with Cathy. I didn't see her before I left. By then all I was thinking about was my baby daughter.

The last thing Dr. Monroe said to me — it was the last time I would see him for many months — "Mr. Beaver, don't expect *anything*. This is just routine to send her to Charlotte. We send all babies like this to Charlotte. Just don't expect *anything*." I didn't have to ask him to repeat himself that time; he had said it clear enough to shoot through even my shock-grogged brain. There was no hope. Routine procedure. End of the drama.

It was very cold when I went downstairs. The lobby was full of people. It's funny how word spreads so quickly when something goes wrong in the hospital. I guess all the orderlies and nurses wanted to see the baby, but they couldn't see anything but an isolette with a lot of blue towels covering the infant's midsection.

I remember saying to the head nurse, "Do these ambulance drivers know what's wrong — just in case something goes haywire?" She had walked down with me to the ambulance entrance.

She didn't answer me. So I asked the emergency attendants, "Do ya'll know what's wrong?"

They said, "No, not really."

I looked at the nurse again. She told them briefly of the situation. Then we were off.

It was about four a.m. in the morning by then. I remember the speed — very, very fast. Flashing lights. No siren. An almost alien environment. I kept trying to talk to the attendant who was driving, afraid that if I didn't talk, I was going to come completely apart. I was crying. Fighting back fear. Overwhelming fear.

I had known fear before — in a car accident or when falling out of a tree or being afraid of being hurt — but I had never known such incredible fear until that ride. It wasn't fear for myself. I was just so afraid that my baby was going to die. For the first time in my life I had something that was a part of me that might slip away before I even had a chance to touch her.

"God, please!" I thought. But God didn't seem to be anywhere in sight.

Satan was. In force. He really moved in. From that point on I don't really remember too much of the ride. Just fear. Overwhelming fear. I knew that my baby was going to die.

Almost silently, we sped towards Charlotte.

5

PAIN, PRESSURE, AND A LITTLE FAITH

BARRY:

Like a zombie, I watched as we arrived at the Charlotte Memorial Hospital emergency entrance. The flashing lights overhead cast an eerie, unearthly glow. I walked beside the isolette as they took it upstairs. Nurses and doctors were already waiting for us.

"What is the baby's name?" an attendant asked, waiting to write the information down.

We hadn't even picked a name out yet. We had thought, Natalie Jean. Or Natalie Deane (after Cathy's middle name). But I didn't want to make the decision there. The lady shook her head and wrote, Baby Girl Beaver. It sounded so cold, antiseptic.

The same lady wanted information, statistics, insurance, addresses. I thought, "Lady, this is so very irrelevant to what's happening. You can get to me anytime." I mean, I wasn't trying to be stubborn or just ignore her, but I wasn't the least bit interested in what she had to say. I was thinking, "Golly, lady, shut up! Let's get the baby up to the doctor."

I think she expected me to stand there, but I just kept on walking. I figured that if she wanted to talk to me, she could walk with me. She did. She rode up in the elevator, asking me questions. I kept trying to answer them as effectively as I could under the circumstances. I still was pretty much in shock.

Actually though, the lady helped provide a break, distracting me for a moment as I began trying to deal with these horrible waves of fear.

When we got upstairs, they immediately took the baby into the Intensive Care Unit. All of the nurses kept going inside to look at her, then they'd look at me.

They had already called Dr. James Hamilton, one of the finest surgeons of his type in the East. He was going to try to stretch the skin and cover the exposed organs.

I felt like a "basket case." The two residents on the floor came out. I was crying in the hallway. They led me to a waiting room. I didn't want to

Pain, Pressure, And A Little Faith

leave my baby, but they knew I couldn't go in where they would be doing surgery, and they felt that I should sit down somewhere. They tried to comfort me, but I was really starting to come apart.

I kept saying to myself, "I've got to hold up. I've got to make it through this — no matter what happens."

But all the time I was crying. All I could think about in my mind was the devil laughing at me — like my hopes and dreams were such futile efforts. "There's no absolutes," he mocked. "You can't plan your life. Even the God-life changes all the time. Things just aren't like you have thought they were. And I can throw a monkey wrench into your life anytime I want to."

I looked at the two young men — "How can this be happening?" I wanted to find somebody to grab and feel like there was at least something I could hold onto. But there was nobody there. Nothing.

The two residents finally had to leave. I wish they hadn't. It really got bad — the pressure.

Dr. Hamilton arrived, but I didn't get to see him. He went in directly to scrub up for surgery. A nurse told me, then took me down to the next floor into a waiting room crammed with other people, a huge corridor-like room. The lights were out. It was around five in the morning by then.

I went in. Sat down. And from that point on, I felt like I went head-to-head with every demon in hell. The worries and fears about my baby were being compounded.

I had never been like this before. Everyone considered me the "Rock of Gibraltar," especially since I had come to the Lord a few years before.

But I was losing it dramatically. I could see a panoramic view of everything wrong I had done in my life — my rebellion in college, the drinking and partying life as a club musician and my failures as a son and husband.

"It's all your fault," I heard. Every Christian wants to do right, especially when he reaches a real level of commitment as I had during the past few years, but each also falls and stumbles and makes mistakes. I had. And Satan poured it on — "You never learn from your mistakes. You'll never overcome your mistakes. Look at you — you think you've grown so much during the past two years. You've gotten involved in this whole 'Holy Spirit baptism' thing, and now your rug is being jerked out from under you. Sure, you've talked about faith, but what good is it doing you now. Ha-ha-ha!" It was torment. Straight from the pits of hell.

I tried to say the name, "Jesus." I knew that the Bible says that at the sound of Jesus' name, the demons flee. Well, I was trying to get his name out, but — unreal — it wouldn't come out too well. I was thinking, "If I could only keep saying the name of Jesus, this torment would leave me a little bit."

But the shock and trauma of dealing with what I saw back there in the Cabarrus Memorial Hospital when Dr. Monroe pulled back the blue towels — the "Rock" kept crumbling. The ride down to Charlotte, the fact that I had nobody to lean on — I was totally crumbling.

I had always considered myself pretty secure, that I could handle things. But I didn't know just how unstable I was — spiritually, physically, or mentally — until those early morning hours.

As I sat there in the surgery waiting room, the battle raged. Fear and doubt in myself as a Christian became mind-throbbing. Intense. I even began doubting that God was real. Satan kept bringing one major thought back to my mind, blasting me with it — "Your baby's messed-up stomach is because of things you did before you became a Christian."

"No!" I cried inside my mind. "No! God doesn't do things like that."

But I doubted my own words. I couldn't feel God with me. That increased the doubt. "Have I fooled myself for the last two years into thinking that I had a real relationship with God? Have I really goofed up so bad that even he doesn't want me?"

I could see daylight coming through the window, but my mind was still shrouded with wave after wave of doubt and fear.

If it is possible to be in the pits of hell without actually dying, I was there that morning. Satan walked all over my faith. He stomped me into a mass of twisted, broken pieces. I felt like a mass of jagged nerve endings. Throbbing. Uncontrollable.

I kept going up to the overseer of the waiting room to see if the surgery was finished and if Dr. Hamilton had come by yet.

By eight that morning, I kept thinking, "It's been three hours. Where is the doctor? I've got to talk to him."

I wanted to be there when the doctor came through — just to hear if my baby was still alive, just to know if there were any chances for her making it. But I also needed to go to the bathroom really bad. I was already dealing with all my doubts, and I thought, "I've got to get out of here. Walk around, even if it's just to the bathroom. I need to hit somebody. Something. I can't take it." I felt like I was fighting some unseen force, and nobody else in the waiting room even knew that it was going on. All they could see were my tears.

When it reached the breaking point, I went ahead to the bathroom. A real battle was going on inside. I kept crying out to God for relief.

Sure enough, during the few brief moments I was in the bathroom, Dr. Hamilton came through, saw I wasn't there and left! It would be

Pain, Pressure, And A Little Faith

three days before I would see or talk to him.

That was the last thing I needed. Already I was bouncing on the bottom of my black emotions, and then that too.

But the time in the bathroom had been a breaking point, of sorts. As I cried out to God, there was a little relief from the frightening waves about to drown me.

When I sat down, I forced myself to begin speaking the name of Jesus. "Jesus... Jesus... Jesus..." I could tell that something was happening. The pressure eased a little. God had moved in on the scene. For the first time, I began thinking straight.

It was just in time. My mother and father arrived then, but we only talked a moment since a nurse came down to take me up to see my baby. Surgery was over.

I had to scrub and put on the sterile surgical garb quickly. My mother and dad were standing there looking through the glass. I could see, as I walked into the room, that it was a very isolated-type Intensive Care Unit exclusively for children.

Fear blasted me again. Maybe it was the fact that I had been up all night. Maybe the alcohol-like smells. I had never seen anything like the room with all the sick children.

I walked over to my baby girl. She was lying there on her back in the isolette. Her tiny arms and legs were taped down so that she couldn't pull anything loose. She had tubes in her nose, IVs in her arms and feet and hands and head. She had a respirator on her. She was lying there trying to cry, but I couldn't hear a sound — just a rasping noise since the respirator tubes going down her nose blocked the larnyx.

My tears came like a flood. I felt so helpless. Just an incredible helplessness. That was my little baby girl, a part of me, and I couldn't do *anything* to help her!

I reached down to touch her, and then the most incredible thing happened. She took hold of my finger. Here was this tiny little thing, just out of surgery, no hope for her survival, and she was squeezing my finger!

I squalled. The situation was so hopeless anyway, that just intensified everything. I was really, really hurting, wishing that there was something I could do. The nurses in the ICU were trying to comfort me, and one — Mrs. Brown — came up and put her arm around me. I must have looked so pitiful, but she looked me squarely in the eyes and urged, "Just have a little faith."

It was so simple, so soft, and yet it was like somebody had just given me a shot of adrenalin or something when she said that.

God truly used that woman and five little words to shock me back into what was going on. I wanted to believe again.

I looked at the nurse. Then I looked back at my baby. I was still crying, but I felt faith welling up

Pain, Pressure, And A Little Faith

in my heart. I could feel Satan's power over me being broken. I began thinking about the healing power of God. It was like her words had brought me back to my spiritual mind, and I felt it coming back strong.

I even said what I was feeling. I looked down at my little struggling girl, and said to her, "Jesus is going to heal you!"

She didn't know what I was saying, of course, but it was spoken as much for me as for her. I kept saying it, "Jesus is going to heal you." I was speaking faith. I felt God expanding inside me.

I looked around at all the equipment and human effort going on in there to save lives, to keep children breathing, and I looked through opened eyes — "Even with this," I thought, "how could anyone survive apart from your healing hand?" It made me more determined in my heart that I was never, never going to let go of my faith in God again.

I had been to the bottom, to the very last inch of a huge black pit, and I didn't like it. I had never had a test of my faith before.

I heard the sounds inside that room with new ears — the monitor machines with the little buzzing sounds. It didn't matter what happened in that room. I had faith. I remembered again God's prophecy over Cathy, "I'll protect you and that which is within you, because I am your God, and I will restore you to perfect health."

For some reason, it didn't even matter when

the head pediatrician admitted, as soon as I left my baby and began taking off the surgical togs, that there was little hope.

It didn't matter anymore that when we had left Cabarrus Memorial during those predawn hours, that my baby's situation was impossible. Forget it. Those kind of cases don't live. Don't expect anything.

I knew once again that man does not have the last say-so.

It's easy to be taught faith, to say it to yourself, to tell others all about it — but until one walks through the valleys, he doesn't know what it's really all about.

It was just a beginning — that morning with our baby, that time when the nurse said to have a little faith — but it let me know how powerful positive words were.

I had talked about confessing the Word of God before, lots of times. That's one thing. It's quite another to be shell-shocked and not even realize for a while what is going on.

It was interesting that the devil knew how powerful the Word of God is. I was losing the battle. I had never had such an attack on my mind. I was going through an incredible, spiritual, mental warfare. I kept losing. I thought, "My God in heaven, what's going on?" I asked, "How can I get through this?" I don't know how I came through it, to be honest.

I had always heard that when a Christian gets

Pain, Pressure, And A Little Faith

to a point where he feels he can't go any farther, physically or mentally, then the line is dawn. God says, "Okay, that's all. There's no more, now. You don't need to go through this anymore. That's enough."

A smart Christian takes those moments and builds on them. When another situation comes up, then the wise believer remembers what he's already been through.

I learned something in the midst of the worst catastrophe. Most people "flake out" as Christians and give up because they can't continue on when they get knocked down. They often just get up long enough to relieve the problem. That's all.

Real faith is enduring. It never gives up, no matter what the scope of the problem is. It never wears out, no matter how faint the believer is.

As for me, I can always go back to that spot in my mind and remember that God solidified my mind there in the hospital that morning. I started at unmerciful fear, and God helped me through. My daughter had no hope, yet he told me that he was in control.

After Mrs. Brown, the nurse, made that statement, the next few minutes God truly began increasing my faith. He began showing me that he was aware of the problem. It was like, "Zap! Barry, snap back. Don't you remember who I am?"

Of course I was still distraught as I remembered my little baby, her body riddled with surgical and life-sustaining equipment, but God's presence moved in. I knew, for the first time, that everything was somehow going to be okay. I just didn't know how. All of my five senses told me otherwise. But God...

6

ALONE TOGETHER

BARRY:

As I walked out of the Intensive Care Unit and prepared to take off the green clothes, it suddenly hit me that I hadn't even thought about Cathy.

I mean, at first, when the nurses and doctors were scurrying about during the birth, Cathy was all I was thinking of. I figured that she was really in trouble. I gave no thought as to the baby's health.

Then, when I found out that our newborn girl was so totally messed up, my thoughts completely switched to the baby. I hadn't even had time to think about my wife back in the Cabarrus

Memorial Hospital.

As I got in my mom and dad's car, no one was talking very much. They were in such shock themselves. We had always been such a close family. My dad had always wanted a daughter — all he got was twin boys (Larry and I). I looked at my dad — "Well, you finally got your little girl ..." We both broke up. Neither of us said anything more — all of us were afraid we'd come completely apart. By the time we got back to Concord and drove into the hospital parking lot, Cathy had long since been back in her room.

CATHY:

It took me a long time to wake up. I was so groggy, but finally I began to make more sense of what my daddy was trying to say.

"Cathy," he kept saying, "I've got to tell you something."

"What did I have?"

His eyes kept searching mine to see if I was ready for what he was going to tell me. "You had a little girl, but there is something wrong with her."

"Daddy!" Ice water ran through my veins. "Is she retarded?" That was the only thing I could think of that could be wrong.

"No."

"Well, what are you talking about, Daddy?" I was still a little out of focus, and I didn't understand what he was talking about — all of her organs being on the outside. It just didn't make sense.

"What time is it, Daddy?"

He told me, "6:15, and Natalie is being operated on right now — the doctors are going to try to put everything back in and stretch her skin over the opening." I still didn't really understand all of it — I had never heard of anything like it before. I couldn't even picture what in the world he was talking about.

But I also realized that it had to be pretty serious for Dr. Monroe to send my baby off immediately and do the surgery like he said.

I started crying — such a fear of the unknown. I had looked forward to that moment for so long — the time every mother-to-be dreams about when she wakes up and the nurses bring in the hungry, squirming little baby — just like in the movies.

But just as I started crying, feeling sorry for myself, still trying to make sense out of the nonsense, I remembered something from Oral Roberts' latest book on unwavering faith.

Something inside me sprang up so strong. I knew that right at that moment the surgeons were working on my baby. Something made me grab daddy's hand — "When are we going to believe that God can do anything like we have been saying all along?" (I had grown up in a Pentecostal home).

Daddy looked back at me — "Right now!" We

began praying then. I never, from that moment, doubted that God had everything under control.

Other people came into the room — mama. Jeff — he was headed for the television taping. Others.

I was already going through a battle in my mind — even though I had settled the faith part — asking, "Why?" Then my cousin said, "Cathy, why in the world would something like this happen to you?"

It sliced through my soul. Inwardly, I was already asking, "God, I've served you ever since I was old enough to know anything. All I have ever known in my entire life has been you. And this has to happen to me? Why? God, I don't understand." It really hit me that a malformed baby should have happened to somebody who wasn't living for the Lord — to sinful people. I just couldn't comprehend a bad thing like that happening to someone trying to serve God. "What did I do to deserve this?"

The room had pretty well cleared out by the time Barry returned.

BARRY:

It was pushing 10 or so that morning when I came rushing into Cathy's room. It had been seven hours since our baby was born.

We cried and hugged. There wasn't much need for words. I do remember saying, "Cathy,

Alone Together

God has our little girl in his hands."

That was all. I didn't go into too many details. I mainly wanted her to rest. No doctor told me to keep things from her. I just sensed that she would be stronger the next day. Then we could sit together and go through some things.

If tomorrow came for our little baby...

7

NO END IN SIGHT

My brethren, count it all joy when ye fall into divers (different) temptations;

Knowing this, that the trying of your faith worketh patience.

But let patience have her perfect work, that ye may be perfect and entire, wanting nothing.

If any of you lack wisdom, let him ask of God, that giveth to all men liberally, and upbraideth not; and it shall be given him.

But let him ask in faith, nothing wavering. For he that wavereth is like a wave of the sea driven with the wind and tossed.

For let not the man think that he shall receive any thing of the Lord.

> *A double-minded man is unstable in all his ways.*
>
> *(James 1:2-8)*

CATHY:

Both Barry and I resolved from the very first morning to speak the Word of faith, to constantly think about only the positive. I began picturing in my mind what I wanted — me at home holding my baby girl.

But I don't think that we really realized how grave the situation was. It would be nice to say that we confessed the Word and immediately our Natalie Deane (we named her the second day) was completely healed and we all waltzed off into the sunset. God knows it wasn't like that. Nothing like that.

She lost almost two pounds immediately after that early morning surgery. Then her body began swelling. She had a big tube going into her stomach, a tube into her lungs through the nose and a glucose IV in her left leg.

Two days after she was born, they had to operate again to put a tube in her jugular vein (hyperalimentation line for her to get strength and gain weight).

Her heart stopped on the third night. Somehow they got it started back.

Every day, it seemed, a new emergency or crisis arose. I had to spend seven days after the birth in the Cabarrus Memorial Hospital, then ten days at home. I literally drove Barry crazy — everytime he would come into my room, I'd beg him to call Charlotte Memorial and ask how Natalie was doing. I asked him again and again to describe what our baby looked like, and felt my heart warm when he talked about her. I had always wanted, always asked God for, a dark-eyed, dark-haired child, and I had always hoped for a little girl.

BARRY:

I was the only link to Natalie that Cathy had. The nurses at Cabarrus Memorial let her use the phone in the nurses' station to call Charlotte and talk to the head nurse in the pediatric ward, but that was hit and miss.

It would be 10 more days even after Cathy got out of the hospital before she could go see her baby. It wasn't for health reasons. The doctors just didn't think that Natalie was going to live a day, let alone a week or more. They were trying to spare her the pain of seeing her baby, getting even more attached, seeing her alive, then the "inevitable" happening. It seemed a foregone conclusion that there was little hope. Even from the beginning, Dr. Monroe (at Cabarrus) had said (in effect), "This is just routine (to send her to Charlotte). Don't expect anything."

Technically, though, Cathy could have gone to

No End In Sight 51

see Natalie very quickly. They were just afraid that when Natalie died (*when* seemed to be the main question), Cathy might snap.

CATHY:

I hardly went out of my room during those seven days at Cabarrus Memorial. My room happened to be the very room across from all the babies — of all places. I told mother, "Why do I have to be stuck here, looking at all those babies out there?"

I kept my door shut all the time. Finally, though, I got up enough courage to go out there — "I'll open the door and go look at the babies in the window."

Something happened inside me, however. My eyes brimmed over with hot tears as I glanced from tiny bundle to bundle. Almost hopefully, I looked for a baby like Barry had described, but I knew that it was just a cruel game — "My baby's not there. I don't want to see them anymore." And I retreated back to the safety of my room.

Another girl on my floor must have been going through the same thing. Her baby had been born with an open spine and was gone. Her door remained shut also. I felt such a kindred compassion, even though I didn't know her, because I knew how she must be feeling. I didn't have my baby either. Only a mother would really understand that. My body had been building up to this moment for months, then . . .

I cried all the time.

BARRY:

We got it worked out so that Cathy could talk at least once a day to the head pediatric nurse in Charlotte. Because of that, Cathy became the main link for information on the days I couldn't get down there. The nursing staff there in Charlotte was so great. I mean, if we wanted to talk five or ten minutes on the phone, they stayed there because they knew what was going on and they really cared.

By the fourth day, Natalie didn't need the respirator anymore. She was able to breathe room air. Her heart seemed fine. She even took a pacifier.

Her bowels began moving too strongly, so the doctors stopped the feeding tube in her neck for a while.

On the sixth day, another victory! They took out the IV from her arm. She didn't need it anymore. She still had the neck (jugular vein) tube and the big tube in her stomach, but she was beginning to grow some.

From that point on (during that first week), I went from the absolute depths of the pits in my mind to the heights of optimism. I was thinking, "Well, I guess we'll have her home in time for

Christmas!" That was only five weeks away, but it seemed feasible to me. "After all," I said, "she's doing so well."

The nurses looked at me like I was some kind of nut. They knew that I had no idea of the gravity of the problem — that the worse was still to come. They were amazed that she was even making it from day to day. Not me! Death wasn't even in the picture anymore. Neither was brain damage or any abnormality.

I think the medical people just went along with me when I talked about taking Natalie home so soon. I distinctly remember Lisa, one of the nurses, looking at me in such total disbelief that I would actually talk about such a thing, but my mind was so fixed that we would have her home quickly that I really didn't realize how bad things were. Or were to become.

November 26, 1975

CATHY:

Natalie was one week old. I left the Cabarrus Memorial Hospital to go home — without my baby. It was such a strange, emotional time. I went out of the corridor in a wheelchair with my suitcases, but no bundle. The worse came when I passed two other mothers who were leaving with their babies safely snuggled in their arms. I couldn't help weeping. It was terrible. Very hard on me.

8

NOT BY SIGHT

CATHY:

Natalie was born on November 19, 1975. I went home from the hospital on November 26. She was one week old. Barry and I had gone through several eternities, or so it seemed.

I mean, we had both made the decision that God was in control, and that we'd both speak faith, but those were spiritual decisions. The natural person in us was a little bit different.

I cried. I'm just very emotional. I'd cry when Barry had to leave in the morning. I'd cry when he came back in the evening. He was trying to get caught up with his work as an insurance representative, but I'm afraid that I didn't help him concentrate on selling policies very much.

I mainly had to lie in the bed. I had labored so long for so many hours without having her that I was really in pain even after I went home. Mother would tend to me. Barry's mother helped take care of me. They were both so good to me. Still, I cried.

Barry couldn't totally fall apart like I did because he had to work. I felt so alone. My baby seemed so far away in some antiseptic-smelling place. I had never been in an Intensive Care Unit before. I tried to imagine what it looked like there, what my little girl looked like.

I had one great fear — I was so afraid that Natalie wouldn't know me as her mother. I mean, all the nurses were taking care of her. It really bothered me — not that they were tending her — but that *I* couldn't. What if she never took to me as her mother?

Two friends of ours also had babies about the same time as I gave birth to Natalie. My mother kept one for the friend one day. The baby's name was Angel. I said, "Let me hold her, Mother."

She looked at me questioningly — "Do you feel like being with a baby, especially since you don't have Natalie here with you?"

"I think I can."

Mama brought Angel into the bedroom where I was lying. I held her, loving on her. I tried picturing myself with my precious little baby that I hadn't even seen yet. But all I could do was cry.

"Mother, come here quick!" I couldn't take it anymore. I wanted it to feel like Natalie, but it wasn't here.

Maybe that's why I kept begging Barry to let me go see my baby. I counted the days.

BARRY:

By the time I brought Cathy home from the hospital, I knew that I had to get back to work. I tried to get down to see Natalie as much as I could, but I also knew that unless I got out selling insurance, she wouldn't have a home to come to.

My business was suffering from a lack of activity. I had totally forgotten about everything. I wanted to concentrate on Natalie and be in constant contact with the people at Charlotte Memorial, but I also had to generate some living.

By the time Natalie was a week old, when I took Cathy home from Cabarrus Memorial, I knew that I had to purposely, against my own will, make Natalie's situation secondary in my mind so that I could function properly, try to do my job and make some sales to get some money coming in.

I think that the basic difference between Cathy and myself on dealing with things—I usually could block stuff out if it was really hard to deal with. I knew that with Natalie, if I didn't keep a guard up properly in battling it, it could almost devastate me emotionally.

Yet, I would let my little daughter's situation still sink in and really get a grip on my mind. I could be driving down the road and not really caring about anything but Natalie, yet I'd also know that I had to make a sale to pay the bills.

I'd stop the car, go in, sit down with the people, and I'd be psyching myself up mentally ("Positive! You're the greatest, Barry! You're gonna sell this one, man!"). But I'd find myself losing track of what I was talking about. We had this dollar guide that my insurance company used to uncover the customer's needs. It was a great program, something that separated the professional from the amateur.

I'd be right in the middle of the presentation, at some particular point, and something would remind me of Natalie. I'd keep talking, but my mind was on the latest crisis, and I'd go completely blank. I don't even want to remember how many times the people would ask me something, and I wouldn't even know where I was or what I was doing.

Cathy didn't understand why I didn't go to the hospital more during those days. My company was putting more pressure on me. Trying to deal with Natalie, dealing with Cathy when I got home, plus getting through the day — it was too much to handle. I'd walk into the house and Cathy would either be real optimistic because she'd heard a good report, or crying because Natalie's condition had reversed.

I was in the worst possible kind of work to try to deal with everything. Being in any kind of sales work is 150-percent attitude. Trying to keep that straight even under normal circumstances is difficult enough without something else.

I lost my appetite. I found out then that if one has so much on his mind all the time, he becomes consumed with those problems. I forgot about living, about everyday life. Nothing else mattered except getting Natalie well. And yet I knew that I had to go on. Somehow.

I made a decision during those dark days. I knew that I had to talk faith and surround myself with faith-talking people. I knew that I couldn't leave even a little bit of myself open to the negative.

I kept being hit with, "Well, if it's God's will for Natalie to die, then you'd be better off."

I didn't need that kind of thing around. From family members. From friends. Nobody.

Cathy and I both sought out people that would encourage us. We knew that God would deliver our little girl.

Positive words. Words of faith. Those were the things that got me through — at work, at home, at the hospital.

Not By Sight

Even when it seemed that Natalie's condition was deteriorating and impossible again and again, we knew that God would restore her. We *had* to walk by faith, and not by sight (2 Corinthians 5:7).

We knew, even from the beginning, that there didn't seem to be any margin for doubt. It drew Cathy and me together. I guess we thought that if we stepped out of line or doubted, God wouldn't have to honor his word in healing Natalie. We were walking softly. We wanted God to know that we were doing everything possible to walk straight in his sight, like, "Look, God, we're doing everything we can do. We want you to heal our baby." I don't think that it was trying to bargain with him, especially since the prophetic word had already come about his protecting and restoring. Mainly, we just knew that we wanted to live a pure life. We didn't want to mess up the miracle that was unfolding.

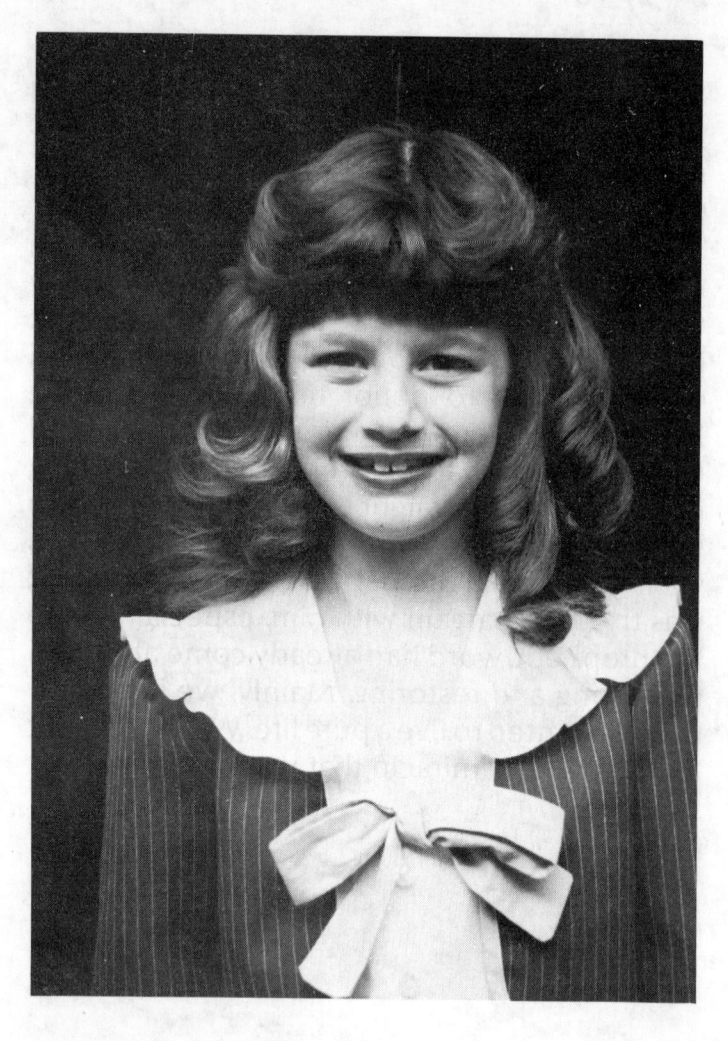

Natalie Beaver — smiling, happy, healthy child. Picture taken in 1984.

Natalie

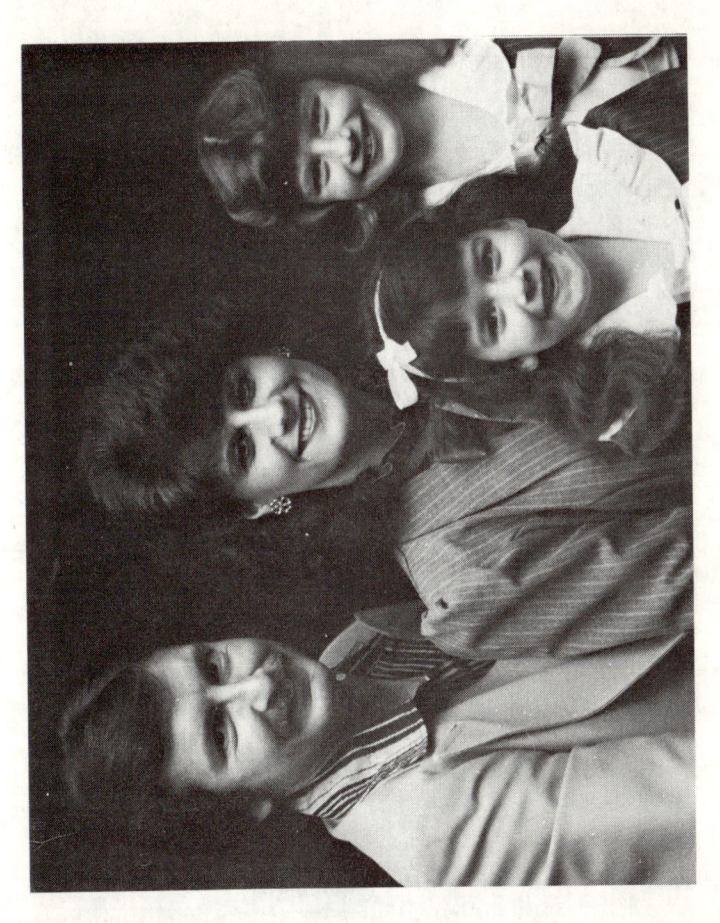

The Beaver family (left to right) Barry, Cathy, Leslie, and Natalie.

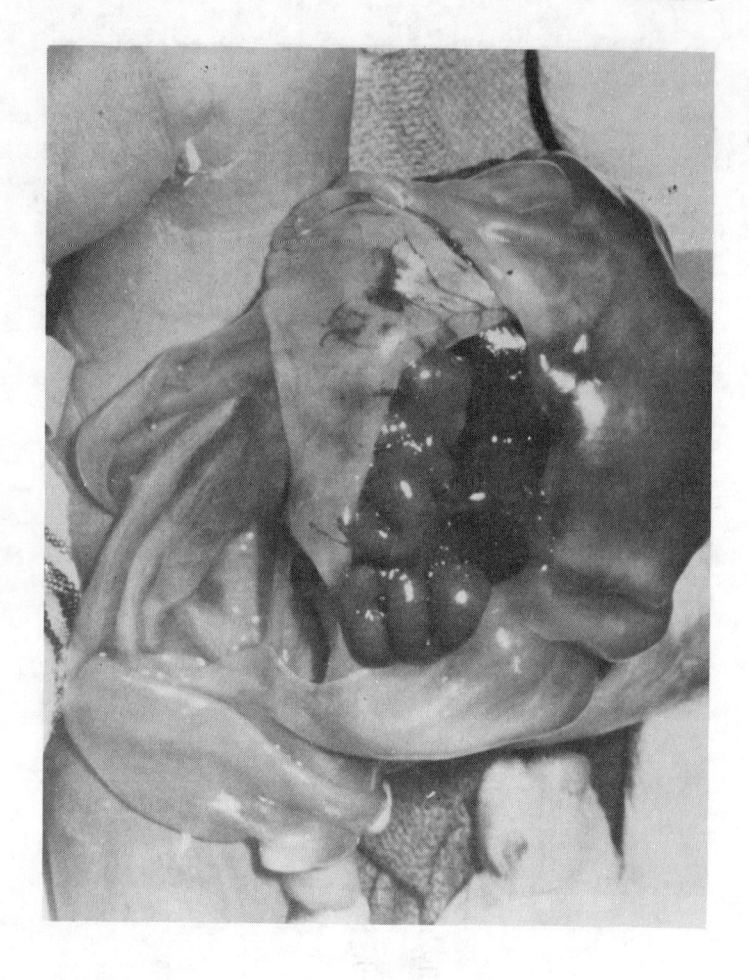

Natalie (before surgery) in Charlotte Memorial Hospital, November 19, 1975, shortly after her birth.

Natalie

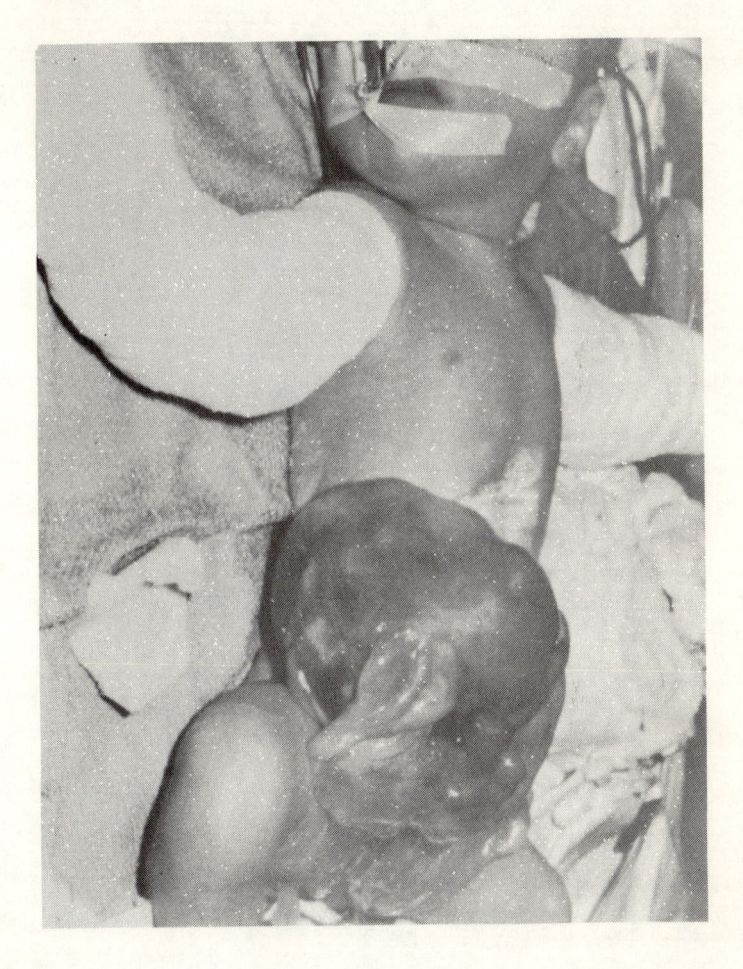

This is another picture of little Natalie, before her surgery.

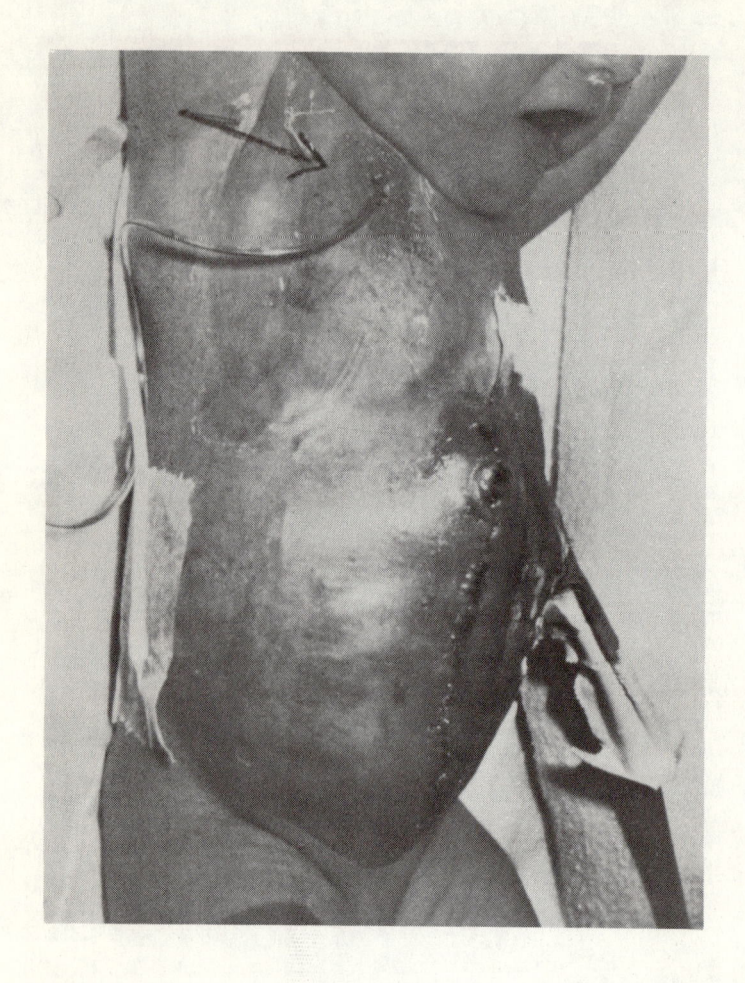

Natalie's frail little body carried this treacherous scar immediately after surgery at Charlotte Memorial.

Natalie

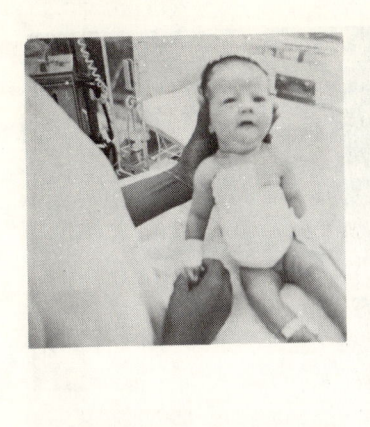

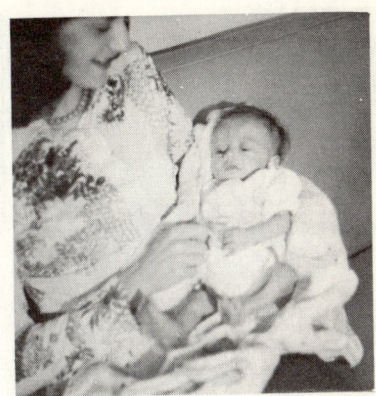

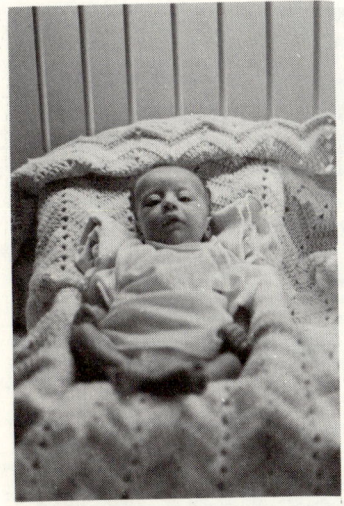

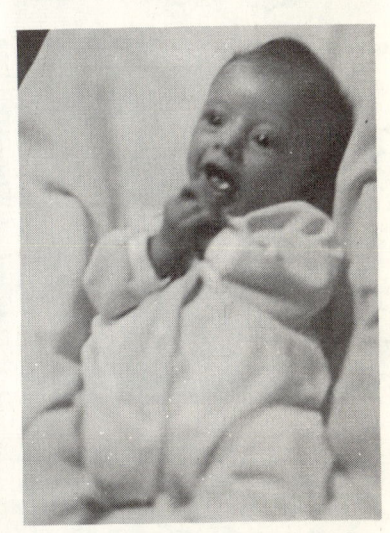

Natalie (upper left) was still in the Intensive Care Unit when she was three weeks and five days old. When she was four months old (upper right) for the first time doctors allowed her outside ICU. Then she was allowed a private room (lower left). Finally, after four and one-half months she was allowed to go home (lower right).

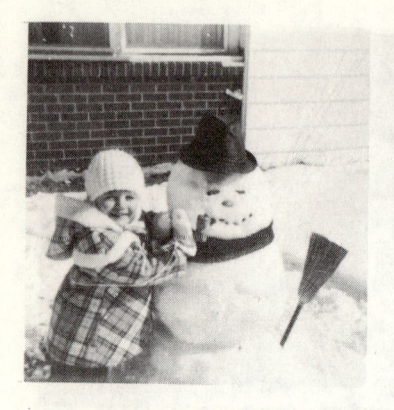

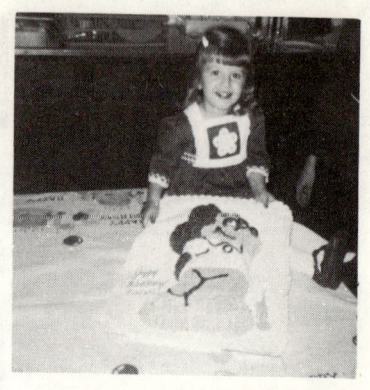

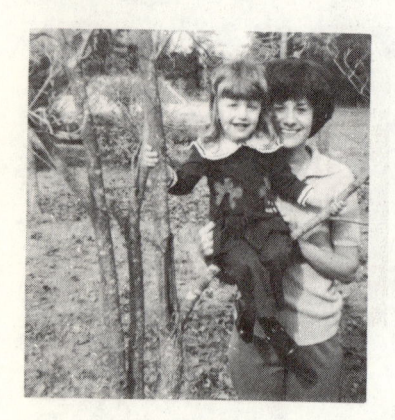

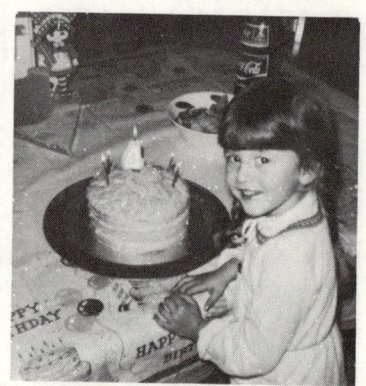

On February 9, 1979, Natalie saw her first snow (upper left). Her third birthday party was a happy occasion for Natalie (upper right). Natalie, age three, and Cathy (lower left). Natalie's fourth birthday (lower right).

Natalie 67

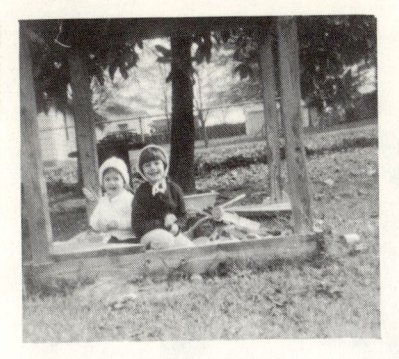

Natalie and Leslie playing in the yard in 1981.

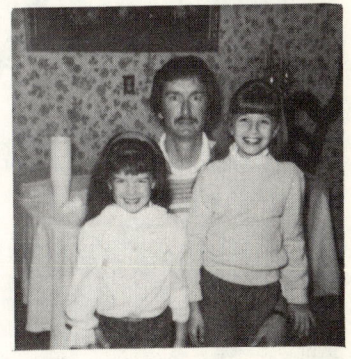

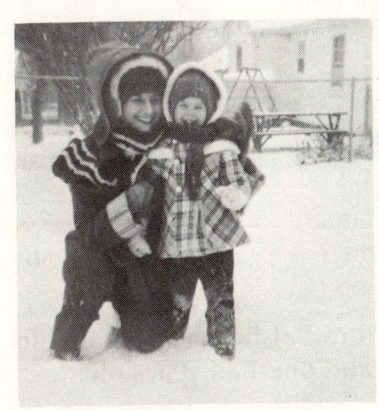

Natalie and Leslie with their father, Barry.

Natalie playing in the snow with her mother, Cathy, during the winter of 1979.

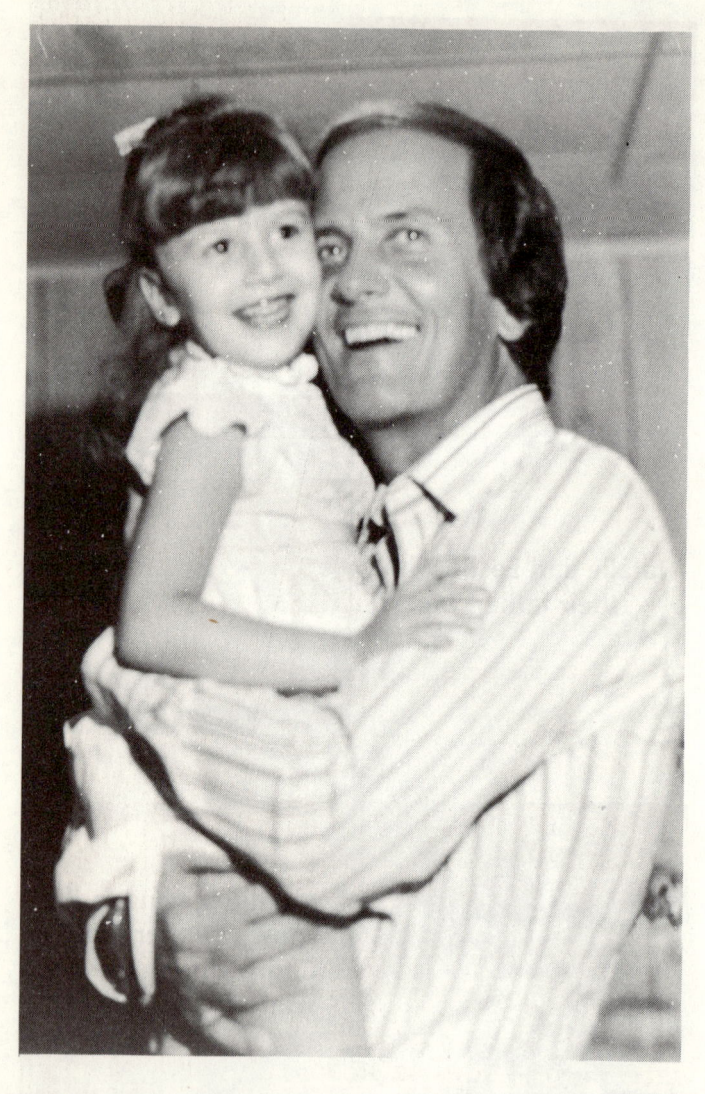

Natalie gets a big hug from Pat Boone. This was in 1981 when she was five and one-half years old.

Natalie

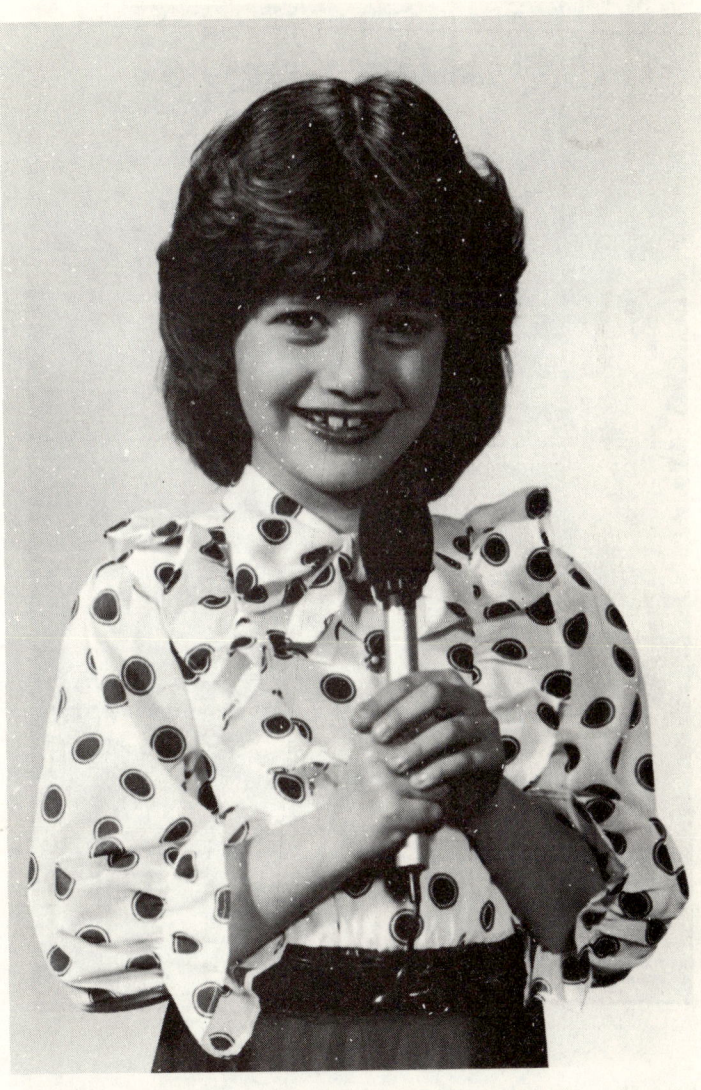

Here, at age seven, Natalie is already a talented and gifted singer.

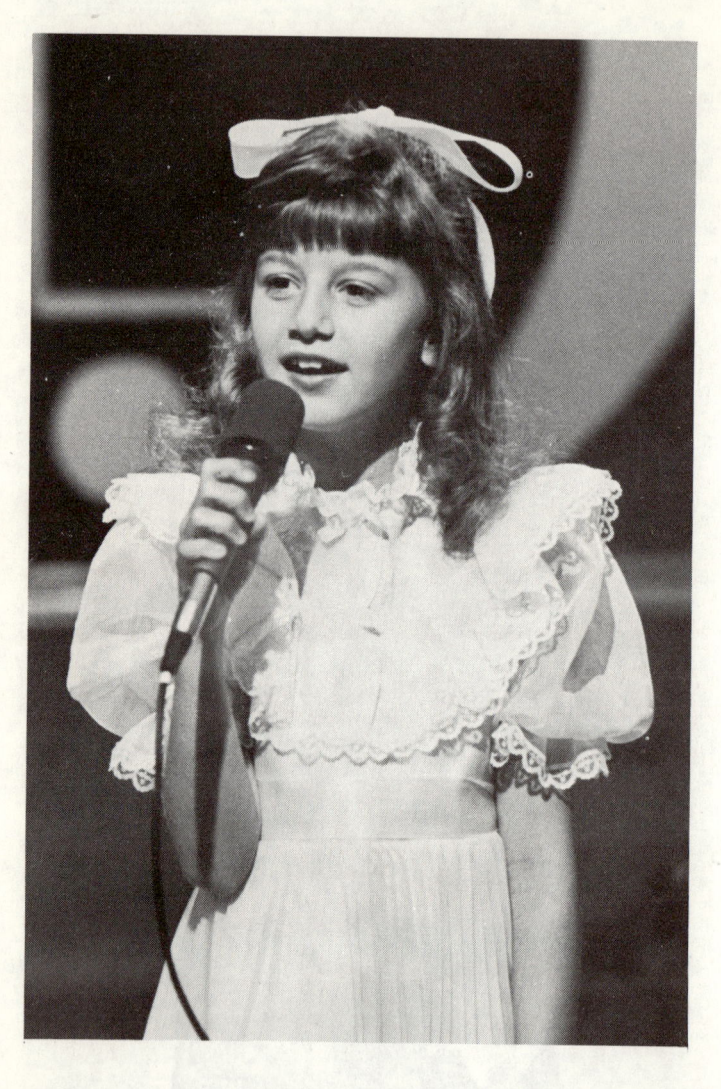

Natalie sang "I'm A Miracle, Lord" on the Jim Bakker Show in September of 1984.

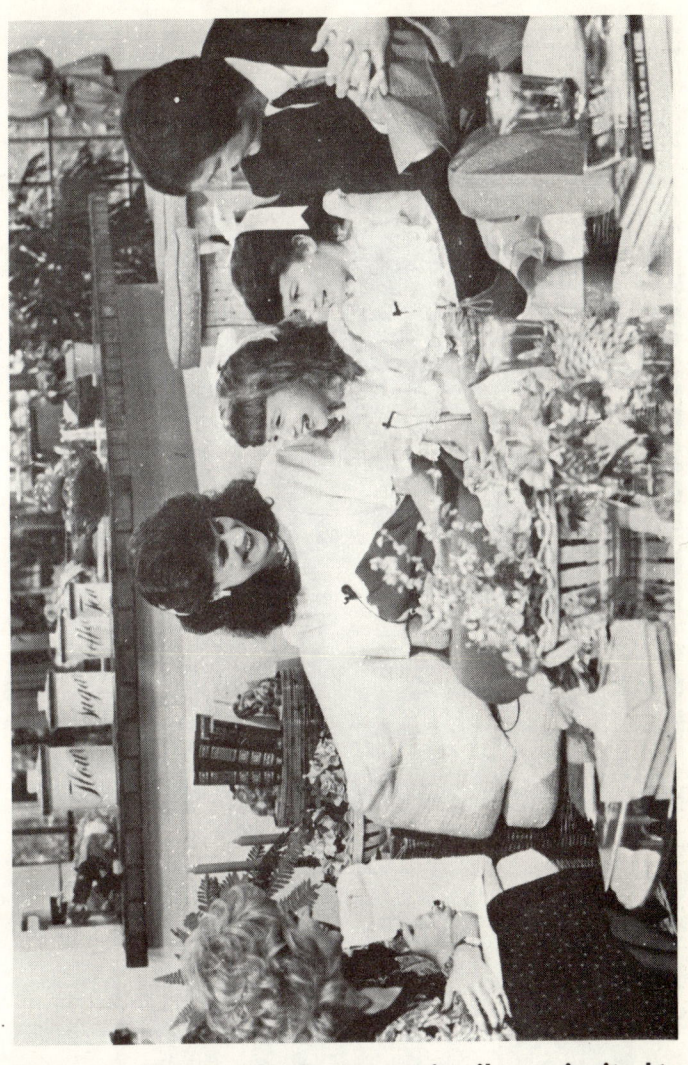

In September of 1984 the Beaver family was invited to appear on the Jim Bakker Show. Here they discuss Natalie's miracle with Tammy Bakker.

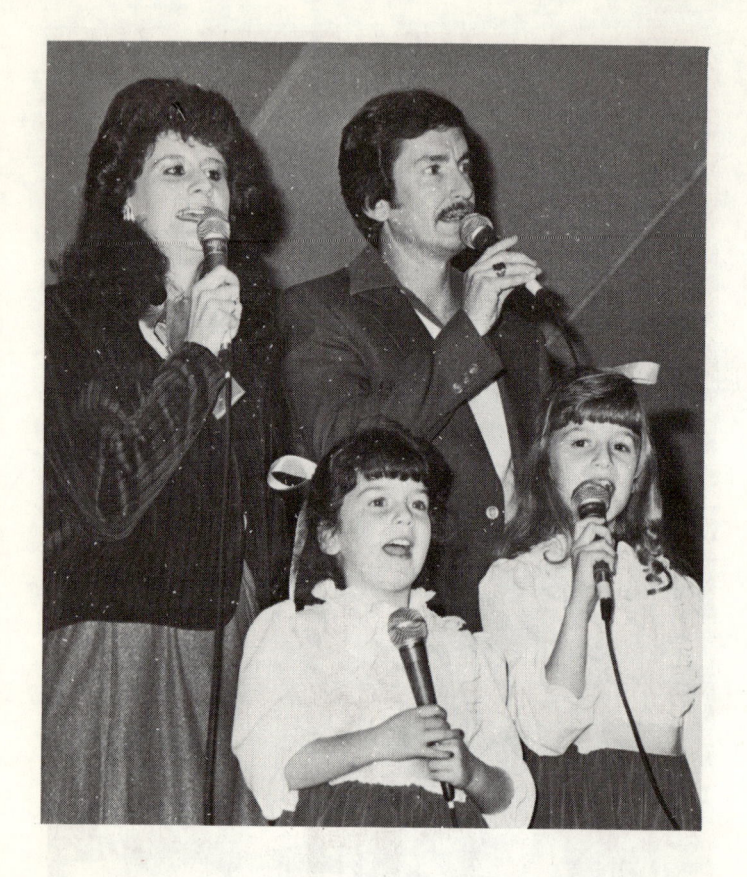

Natalie sings with the family at the PTL Country Fair in October of 1984.

Natalie

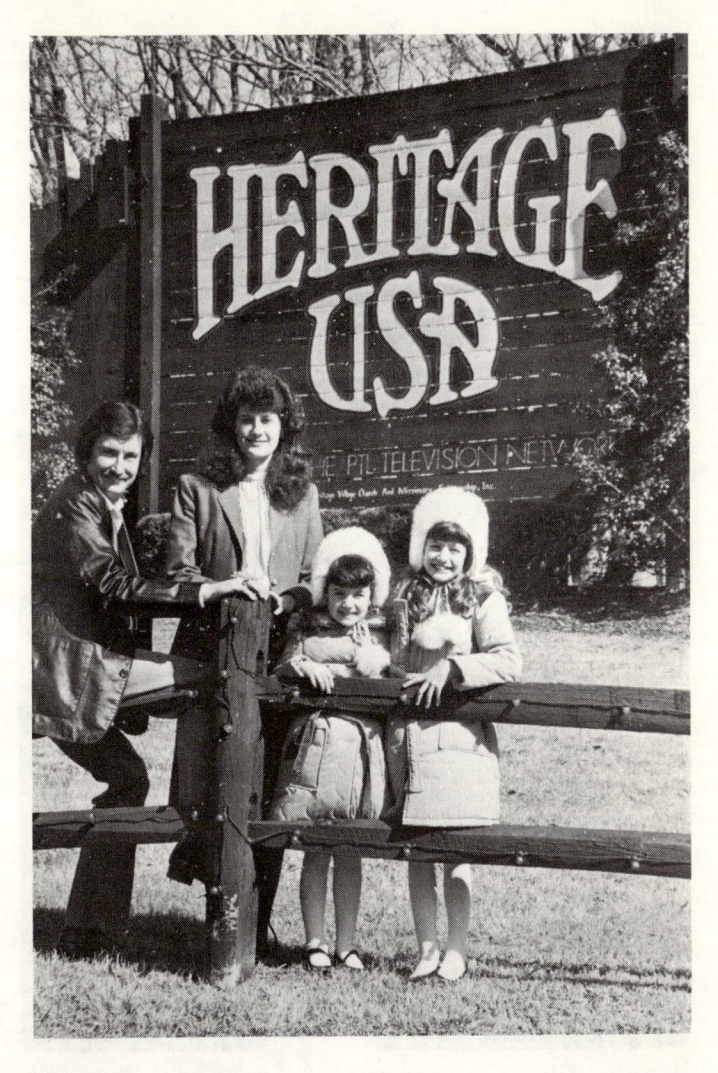

The Barry Beaver family at PTL's Heritage USA in 1985. They are (left to right) Barry, Cathy, Leslie and Natalie.

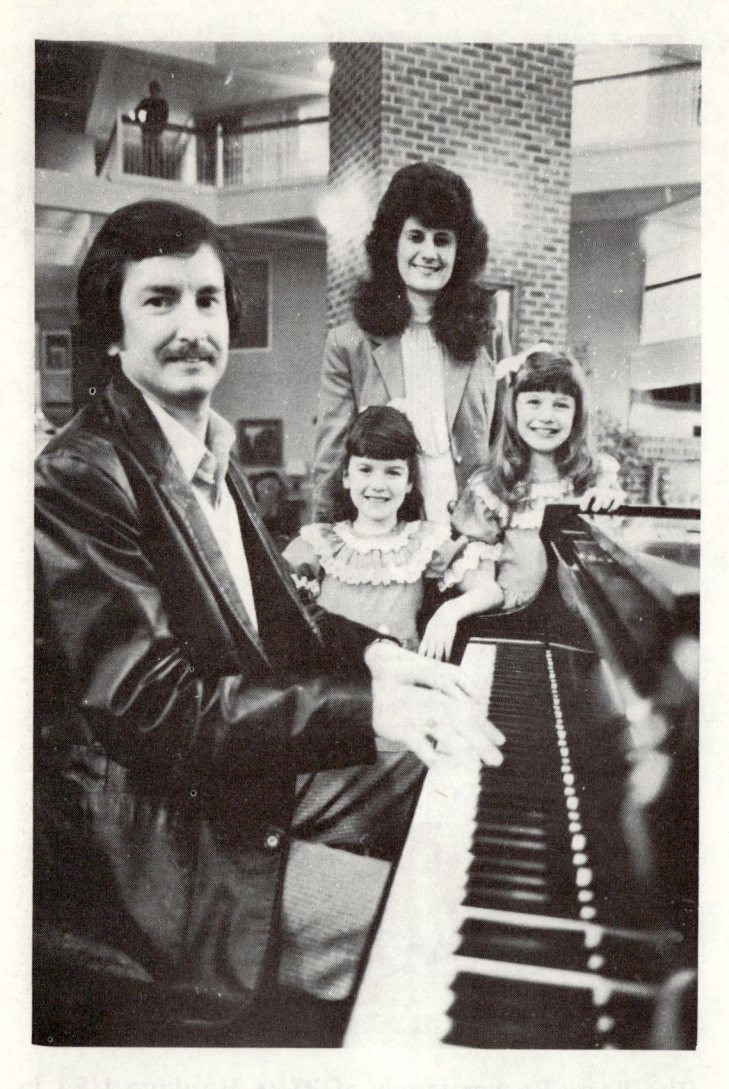

The Beaver family sings together at PTL's Grand Hotel in 1985.

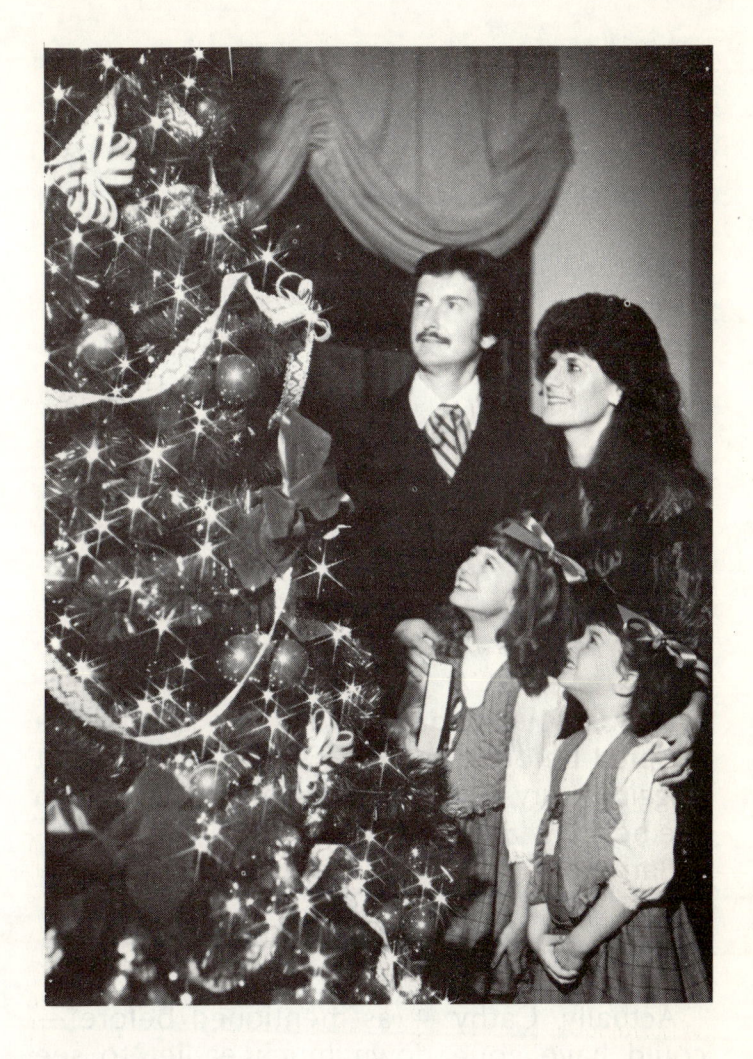

This is the Beaver family as seen on the cover of PTL's *Heritage Herald,* **Christmas week, 1984.**

9

EMPTY BED

CATHY:

It was several days after I got out of the hospital before I could go see Natalie. I kept begging Barry — "I'm getting better. I want to go see her."

Barry said, "No, you have to wait 10 days."

BARRY:

Actually, Cathy — as mentioned before — could have gone down much earlier to see Natalie, but the doctors didn't want her to get attached to the baby. They weren't sure that our daughter would even survive a day, then two,

Empty Bed

then a week. 10 days — it seemed like an impossibility. Why, there were babies coming in with just one organ malfunction who were dying.

CATHY:

On the 10th day we got up early. I couldn't wait to get down to the Charlotte Memorial Hospital. The 30 or so miles seemed like an eternity. Off the interstate. The Charlotte streets wound around. My heart was pounding as we drove into the big circular drive.

When we came to the Intensive Care Unit, I said, "Barry, let me pick her out. Let me pick her out by myself."

But I couldn't find her. I didn't know which one she was. Finally, Barry pointed her out to me. I will never forget that moment. Immediately I began crying really hard. She was so little. I thought, "Dear God, how can she live? She is so tiny."

I cried and prayed as I stood there. I really couldn't believe I was finally seeing my baby. It was *my* Natalie lying there. The tears just fell in torrents.

Cathy's Diary
Dated November 29, 1975 — Saturday

The first time I ever saw Natalie. It had been

10 days. She was so beautiful. So much pretty black hair. Long feet. She weighed five pounds, one ounce.

She opened her eyes when I talked to her. I told her I loved her — that her mama was there.

She opened her big blue eyes and smiled three more times at Barry and me.

We were only allowed 10 minutes inside the unit there with our green uniforms on.

Everytime I'd start to leave Natalie, she would squeeze my hand real tight and look at me. I couldn't bear to leave her. Finally, I had no choice. It was like ripping me away — my heart was still there with my little bundle.

November 30, 1975 — Sunday

Barry and I got to hold Natalie for the first time ever. We were so happy. We talked to her non-stop, telling her, "We love you, baby. Jesus loves you." She quit crying when I rubbed her little back. She smiled at us.

The nurse said that the doctor kept taking pictures of Natalie's stomach. No one can understand how it is holding together.

November 31, 1975

Natalie's weight was up to five pounds and four ounces. My brother (Jeff Wood) and

Empty Bed

Michele (his wife) took me to see her today.

CATHY:

If I went down there, it consumed a lot of my day. It kept my mind off my loneliness and Natalie's problems.

If I left about eight or nine in the morning and got back about three, my whole day was just about over by then. I thought, "If I can just see her, I can get through each day."

Every day I longed to go. I just thrived on it.

BARRY:

Cathy hunted for people to take her down to Charlotte. We had two cars before, but I had sold one just before Natalie was born. Since I had to use it out selling insurance, Cathy had to get people to help her. At the time, her mother didn't have a car to use during the day, but later Thurman bought Phyllis her very first car.

CATHY:

Barry's mother could take me sometimes. A lot of people at our church did too. I would say, "I declare, I wish I had a car to go down to Charlotte tomorrow." They would often say, "Oh! Let me take you." Sometimes at first I had to miss seeing her a day or two, but after my mother got her car, I never missed a day.

Cathy's Diary
December 10, 1975 — Wednesday

The doctor said she is doing well, feeding sugar water through the tube in her stomach — 30 cc's every two hours.

But the nurse said she was getting dehydrated because Natalies's urine was too concentrated. That's why the sugar water was started.

They raised the food level in her chest tube also, hoping she'll gain weight a little faster.

December 14, 1975 — Sunday

She is three weeks, five days old today. Barry and I went to see her and took pictures. She weighs six pounds, two and one-half ounces. She had torn her stomach open nearly all the way except for a few stiches at the bottom and top of her stomach.

We saw it when they dressed her. It was all yellow inside. I didn't see any of her organs showing. They are trying to hold it together with tape.

They said that the skin will have to heal over "somehow." Lisa, a nurse, said it will make a bigger scar since it split open.

There's no infection or pus or redness. That's what they've been looking for. She has none of

Empty Bed

those things. They say it is clean-looking.

CATHY:

About that time, a word came forth during a church service — "My daughter, you've been faithful to me. Did I not promise you that I would be faithful to you? I've heard the cries of your heart. Now lean on me."

The very next day, when I went to see my baby, she was tearing apart worse. It looked horrible — to the natural eye, at least. I couldn't keep from crying. But I remembered what Jesus spoke to me the night before — "Lean on me." I knew I had to.

The main thing — my faith never wavered about this — was that I knew I'd someday bring her home. I never doubted that for a moment. I believed it with all my heart.

In fact, the very first time I went to church — just a couple of weeks after her birth — I got up in front of the church. I told everything I knew that the doctors had told us. Then I surprised everyone by saying, "One day I'm gonna come back in here with my baby, and I'm going to testify what God has done. You're all going to see her." Then I started crying and went to sit down.

Cathy's Diary
December 15, 1975 — Monday

Called the hospital. Lisa, the nurse, said Dr. Hamilton came by today. The skin is holding at the bottom and at the top. The skin will eventually cover it all.
Said they were going to feed her in a couple of days through the tube in her stomach.
Her bowels haven't moved in two or three days. They hope when they start feeding her through the tube, they'll start moving.

December 17, 1975 — Wednesday

Natalie is one month old today! Barry, Jeff, Michele and I went to see her. She slept the whole time but squeezed both our fingers real tight when we would try to leave her. The doctors said that when she is six months to a year old, they'll have to do surgery on her stomach to cover the opening. And when I bring her home I'll have to keep it bandaged. Said that tomorrow they'll start feeding her through the tube.
She really looked beautiful today.

December 18, 1975 — Thursday

Barry called the head nurse at the Intensive Care Unit. They started feeding her through the stomach tube.

If all goes well, they'll start feeding her the milk orally in about two weeks.

Also, the hyperalimentation line in her neck area will come out in a few days.

Her bowels moved today. And the nurse said that the stomach was healing from the inside out — that she will not have to have surgery!

The tube will be left in her stomach a month after we bring her home.

December 22, 1975 — Monday

Barry, Mama, Daddy and I went to see Natalie. She was crying when we came — they had just taken her hyper line out of her neck.

Her head was shaved again and she had a needle in her head to give medicine and liquid in until she can take milk by mouth a lot.

Well, today she took milk. We all got to see her take the bottle for the first time. We cried — just praised God for such a miracle. She just burped and held the milk down without throwing it up. They said they were just going to feed her by mouth from now on.

I got to hold her. She kept looking at me. She's so beautiful. The doctors now say that her organs are working just fine — the bowel movements too.

CATHY:

I wanted to hold her so bad, but it was some time before they would let me. They had so many tubes in her. I wondered, "How can I hold her with all those things sticking out of her?"

Finally, though, when they would give her to me, I would just sit real still in the chair. I was so scared that something would come undone.

But when I went every day, I became impatient waiting and waiting for the nurses to come around and get her out for me. One day, one said, "Do you think you know how to get her out?" I said, "Yes, I'll *learn* to get her out!"

I did, too. I'd go in there and pick her out, but I had to be real careful because the little tubes had to come out right. I'll never forget. I would rock her back and forth, real slow. I would just talk to her a "mile a minute" because I was so scared that Natalie wouldn't know me. That continued to worry me — that she wouldn't know me as her mother. Every time I was there I would talk to her, just talk to her like she was a grown-up child. I guess I was mainly trying to convince her that she was mine.

I'd say mushy things — "Mama loves you. You know mama loves you." And I'd pray for her — "In the name of Jesus, I confess this child's body healed. In the name of Jesus, you *are* healing this child's body, and I'm going to take her home soon." I said that each time I went. If I would put

Empty Bed

her back down, and she would start crying, I couldn't leave her. That was very hard for me.

I'd say to myself, "I'll stay until they ask me to leave." The notice on the door indicated a 15-minute limit, but I'd sit in that rocking chair and say, "God, please just let them let me stay." Sometimes I'd stay in there one and one-half hours. I figured that as long as they didn't say anything, I was going to stay.

BARRY:

I kept thinking that Natalie would be able to come home by Christmas. The nurses and doctors looked at me with such disbelief when I confessed that. My mind was so fixed on her coming home that I didn't really realize how bad things were. We wanted her home by Christmas — that was our goal.

That she would live — that was already assumed. We didn't even question that, even though the medical people still did.

But as happens many times, our timetable wasn't God's. Natalie spent Christmas in the Charlotte Memorial Hospital, not at home.

CATHY:

Because the unit was so germ-free, we couldn't take any presents or Christmasy things in, except a little music box (the nurses had to even disinfect that too).

One of the nurses did loan us a small plastic tree so we could at least take a picture. That was all she could have of her first Christmas.

When I'd have to leave, I would always wind up her music box. When I would walk out, I'd look back at her. If she was crying, I just couldn't bear to leave. A lot of times I would go back in there and pat her because I couldn't stand it.

They said that Natalie didn't cry much — that really hurt me. I knew that she had never known anything but all tubes and pain. Nothing normal like most other babies. It was so sad to me that she had gotten used to it and wouldn't cry much anymore.

Cathy's Diary
December 23, 1975 — Tuesday

I called today. The doctor said there was some bacteria on the specimen they took today. They don't know if it was when they pulled the catheter out, and it was on the tip of the catheter, or if it was floating in her body.

They are giving antibiotic shots to fight this off. I'm just trusting Jesus that there's no infection.

December 24, 1975 — Wednesday

The doctor is going to do a spinal tap on Natalie today. Says it's routine. They are still checking the bacteria. The bacteria didn't grow from the hyper line. They know that now. That's a miracle — if the bacteria had gotten into the main vein, it would have killed her almost immediately. Praise God for that miracle.

Today we took pictures. Her first Christmas. No one really thought she'd last a day or a week, much less until now! It's a little sad to us that all she can have for Christmas is that little plastic tree and her music box, but at least she is alive and growing!

She had a slight yellowish look in her eyes.

BARRY:

There were a number of things that kept showing up wrong with Natalie — things that we sometimes didn't even know about until after the crisis was passed.

One was a little black sore on her leg when her calcium level got messed up.

CATHY:

That really worried me. I kept asking the nurses and doctors about it all the time.

They would look at me and say, "Mrs. Beaver is crying again." It was true. Only they didn't know that I was crying *and* praying.

I'd pray when I first got there in the morning, and I'd pray just before I left. I felt so helpless.

It's like she was my child, sure, but I had no control over what was done to her or with her. I was, in fact, only her mother for less than an hour a day. It was the most helpless feeling in the world.

BARRY:

One time Cathy was in Intensive Care, and the doctor came through. He said to the nurse, "Did you give Natalie her heart medicine?" Needless to say, Cathy was totally taken aback. "Heart medicine?" she asked. "Is Natalie on heart medicine?"

"Well, yes," the nurse said, "she's been on it since she was born and had that cardiac arrest!"

We had been told that her heart had stopped, but we didn't know that she was on heart medicine. That scared us. Really! We had thought all along that that crisis was over, at least. But then we were being told that it was a condition still being treated.

It seemed like everytime we went in, there was something else wrong with our baby.

Cathy's Diary
December 31, 1975 — Wednesday

Today she was six weeks old. She was more yellow-looking, but the nurse said that she wasn't sick.

They did run tests on her liver and said there seemed to be an abnormality.

January 1, 1976 — New Year's Day

Barry, Mr. and Mrs. Beaver, and I went to see Natalie. The doctor came by while we were there. He said she did have some abnormality in her liver since they had put it back inside her.

She vomited while we were there.

January 5, 1976 — Monday

Barry called the hospital this morning. The doctor said the liver test results would be there tomorrow morning. He said they were feeding her every two hours.

January 6, 1976 — Tuesday

She's still looking yellow. The doctor is discussing whether to do a biopsy on her liver. Said there is something abnormal. They won't be able to give her anything to go to sleep during the biopsy because it's so strong.

My God will take care of her because she's his.

January 7, 1976 — Wednesday

Natalie was asleep when Barry and I got there. Peggy, one of the nurses, changed her bandage while we were inside. It really looked better — not as big a gap. The skin has grown together some. It's not a big lump like it used to be. She's still as yellow-looking; plus, Lisa (the nurse) said that Natalie spit up all her feedings today.

January 8, 1976 — Thursday

They still don't know if a liver condition is causing jaundice. Dr. Hamilton doesn't want to do a biopsy unless it's really necessary.

The doctor said that her liver condition could be from pushing the liver and all her organs back inside during that first morning's surgery.

BARRY:

It was interesting that some of the problems which began to crop up were possibly related to Natalie's first morning's surgery.

When she had first began to come out of Cathy, Dr. Monroe had rushed to grab a big plastic bag. He let Natalie plop into it as she was born.

Then, when they placed her into the isolette, she was all over the place.

When she arrived at Charlotte, the doctors just tried to get all her organs back inside in some general order. They knew that the longer she was all apart, the greater risk of infection.

Plus (and quite honestly), the operation was more a technicality than anything. No one, at that point, expected Natalie to survive. It was preposterous for her to live. There were babies that just had one organ messed up who died. Natalie had them all out.

The liver problem started cropping up. They could see that the situation was never getting any better — "Expect this baby to have liver problems all her life."

We couldn't believe that God would bring her through everything just to get worse.

I think the single most important thing which carried me through this thing was that I searched for people who would speak in a positive way. Cathy and I would both go out of our way to be around people like that. It became the driving force.

We would be somewhere telling somebody what God was doing for our baby. Maybe I wouldn't be feeling so "gung ho" or full of faith at the time, but something I'd say would trigger a faith button in them. Often the other person would come back with something like, "Well, praise God, brother! There isn't a devil in hell who can defeat you." It was like something I really needed at the time — the same for Cathy. Those faith words would just pour out, and we would become like sponges soaking them up. Soon we'd feel like an invincible Spanish Armada, knowing that our faith could fight off anything.

Most of the people who went to our church were faith-building people, so they didn't give us much negative feedback.

Some people we knew did — the negative talk. I mean, even after Natalie had made it through all the stuff during those first weeks and months, everytime something else popped up — like the liver problem — we'd start hearing the "well-maybe-it's-God's-will-that-she-go-on-to-heaven" junk!

But we had to admit that it looked serious — the liver problems. Jaundice to most parents is nothing. Most little babies born are jaundiced for a little while. The main thing about Natalie's was that cirrhosis was setting in, and her liver just wasn't functioning properly.

Cathy's Diary
January 9, 1976 — Friday

Mother and I drove over to see Natalie today. We got there just as Mrs. Mason, the nurse, was giving her 10 a.m. feeding.

Natalie noticed me — those big eyes just looking at me. Then, as Mrs. Mason laid her down, I held my baby's hand and rubbed her little head. She never cried at all. Her milk went down the stomach tube and stayed.

She weighs six and one-half pounds today. The nurse said that she hardly ever cries. She just looked at me the whole time. I played her music box a lot for her.

Her eyes are deep blue-green. She's still

Empty Bed

looking yellow.

January 11, 1976 — Sunday

Barry and I went to see Natalie today. She was awake when we got there. Bad news! She threw up all the night before. Plus, there's a rash on her bottom. The hole where her stomach tube is has been draining some.

I got to feed her in bed. She really wanted her milk. Barry got to burp her and hold her.

He just loved it. Her eyes were so pretty and bright as her daddy held her.

We talked to the doctor. He said they planned to do a biopsy on her liver in a few days. The doctors want to see why she's had jaundice for so long and what's wrong with her liver.

January 13, 1976 — Tuesday

Jeff and Michele took me this morning to see Natalie. I brought her to the window for my brother and sister-in-law to see. They were changing her stomach bandage, so they got to see her stomach. It really is looking good, at least to me. It is granulating (a covering, of sorts). I got to hold her. She fell right asleep. Has held food down since Sunday. Praise my precious Jesus!

January 14, 1976 — Wednesday

They did a biopsy today at 5:15 p.m. It took only a few minutes. The piece of liver was black.

Dr. Hunt did the biopsy. They had plasma going in and an IV in the top of her foot.

She has lost down to five pounds and 14 ounces. Also, Dr. Hamilton suspects hepatitis is causing her to not hold her food well.

When will it end? It seems like one thing piling up on top of the other.

We are anxiously awaiting the report of her liver biopsy.

BARRY:

We went home and prayed. Others joined with us. When we went back, her problems just started going away. There was no medical reason for the sudden change. Her eyes began clearing. The yellow just *went!* The jaundice was gone — just like that.

CATHY:

And yet they kept telling us that they didn't know whether her organs were going to function properly.

The real reason they didn't tell us a lot about each problem that cropped up — they weren't

Empty Bed

trying to keep us in the dark — they were primarily just trying to keep up with each new situation which threatened her life. Everytime they would run a blood test, by the time they would find out what was wrong, those symptons would be gone (or healed), and something else would be happening.

BARRY:

We looked in her eyes. That's always one of the places to tell if a person has bad liver trouble — the whites of the eyes turn yellow. Hers were like that from Day One.

Then, within just a few days, the yellow was gone. It didn't just gradually go away. The doctors were astounded.

"God," I said, "we have believed and now you have let us see it in the natural. We've been hanging onto the supernatural for so long, and you've now even brought it down so our five senses could take it in."

The healing of the jaundice and liver problems were a catalyst in my mind. I knew then that she was on her way out of that place.

And it was a real turning point in my mind as far as *seeing* what my heart had been telling me all along. I could see it happening to Natalie. I could look at her and tell.

But, of course, the problems were not over. Far from that. In some ways, they were just beginning.

CATHY:

I don't think we really knew just how bad Natalie's liver problem was until after it was over.

I mean, we knew that she had jaundice and liver difficulties.

But one day, not long after Natalie's yellowness went away dramatically, I was in with Natalie. A nurse came by with a little group — they looked like student nurses — and the nurse was telling them about Natalie. She said, "This is the baby that had cirrhosis of the liver."

My head jerked towards her — "Are you talking about Natalie?"

"Yes," she said, "this is the child they said that had cirrhosis of the liver."

Well, it was the first time I had ever heard that.

We just had to let them keep doing what they knew to be best for her.

And we kept praying. God had brought us this far.

BARRY:

We just projected the best in our minds. We saw her continually getting better. In fact we saw her well and going home — even during the darkest valleys. We took pictures of Natalie during those times, and our friends and relatives

Empty Bed

looked at the pictures — they couldn't believe how pitiful she looked. Cathy and I thought they were great pictures. We didn't even know how bad Natalie looked because we had projected and imagined that our baby was okay instead of how dire the situation was.

Maybe that was one of the reasons God blessed us like he did. Even with the problems to come.

Cathy's Diary
January 16, 1976 — Friday

The doctor told us he couldn't ask for a better report on Natalie's tests. Her liver is normal! Her feedings are going better. Praise God!

January 17, 1976 — Saturday

Barry and I went to see our baby. She was awake and had those eyes looking all around. I said, "Hello, Darling!" She smiled.

She spit up two times today. But at least her stomach is almost all closed together. It looks fantastic. A scab is forming, but the doctor keeps pulling it off so germs won't get under it.

The nurse still said that she'd probably have problems all her life with her liver, but we know better. God has given her great health!

January 20, 1976 — Tuesday

Natalie's wound has completely shut up now. It's still draining a little bit.

The nurse has now told us that Natalie can come home when she can hold her food down all the time.

CATHY:

God honors the determination of a Christian's faith. There are testing times in everyone's life to see if that person has what he really professes to have.

But through all those testing times, Jesus works out patience and helps us exercise our faith more and more. All those trials which come can build and mold the spiritual man inside.

When things go smooth, we don't have to look up quite so often to say, "God, where are you?"

But just as soon as a test comes — sickness or whatever — we begin seeking his face and asking why it's happening to us. We began getting into his Word to find answers. And the answers are always there.

All Jesus wants us to do is simply look upward and say, "Lord, I believe — no matter what things look like — I still believe."

When things look the worse, that's the very time when God seems to turn things all around.

Empty Bed

BARRY:

And the very moment we'd begin to say, "I just can't hang on much longer and believe— nothing is happening, even though I'm trying to believe with all that I have inside me."

But we should never give up. We knew that we had to keep on believing— keeping hanging on — never quitting in our believing.

Cathy's Diary
January 25, 1976 — Sunday

Barry and I went to see our baby. We both got to hold her during her two o'clock (afternoon) feeding.

A little milk came out the bottom of her tube. She slipped back down to five pounds, 11 ounces because last night she threw up three times.

Her stomach really got tight Saturday night, they said, so they're going to put an IVAC machine to the tube in her stomach like an IV would be in her arm, but there is no needle since the tube is already there. The milk will just drip all day long.

She really cried when she thought we were leaving. One time she just clutched my hand against her chest.

I kept rubbing her head and she finally fell asleep. Then we had to leave.

January 27, 1976 — Tuesday

Mama and I went to see Natalie. I stayed about an hour and a half. She was smiling in her sleep. The doctor said her stomach was still tight, and said if she'd gain some weight that it would loosen it.

I just held her and talked away. She just listens to me, then goes to sleep. I'm so thankful for our God giving her to us.

January 28, 1976 — Wednesday

She has thrush in her mouth — there's no pain to it, just a white coating in the roof of her mouth and on her tongue.

They are giving her medicine for it — drops in her mouth.

January 29, 1976 — Thursday

The thrush is making her little mouth tender. The nurses are having to hold her more to keep her from crying so much.

The thrush is caused by bacteria.

BARRY:

I guess the worse thing, day after day, was the unbearable tension. Pound...pound...pound. It seemed like one thing would go wrong, then

God would heal that. Another thing would go wrong. Always the danger of something going badly for Natalie.

It was like having no appetite after a while. It was always on my mind. It's like almost forgetting about living because I was so consumed with the problems always cropping up.

It's like nothing else matters or has any importance. Yet we had to keep surrounding ourselves with faith-talking people.

The more positive talk we got really helped. Then, after so long, we would get numb to the tension. Somehow, as the weeks turned into months, we sort of got used to it. We had to deal with the tensions and anguish every day. It became just a part of our life.

And deep-down, I think it was already settled that we both knew God was going to deliver our little girl.

But we just couldn't escape the tension.

CATHY:

I didn't have a job. Barry at least got to go to work and kinda get his mind off it. My mind really never got away from the situation.

I stayed at mama's during the day, and I tried to go see Natalie every day, but sometimes I just couldn't. Sometimes it would be three or four days because I didn't have someone to take me.

So, I cried. I could always get rid of my frustrations by crying.

Barry dealt with it differently. He said, "Cathy, I can't live in that realm all the time. I would go crazy."

But it worked for me. It was a release valve. I would cry and pray and read my Bible. Mother and daddy would talk to me. That always helped.

Cathy's Diary
January 31, 1976 — Sunday

Barry and I talked to Dr. Hamilton today. He said they're going to put her out in a private room in a few days, and if she continues to do well on her feedings, she can come home soon. They want me to learn how to feed her before that time.

God just keeps answering prayers!

February 2, 1976 — Tuesday

The scab on her stomach opening came off today. The nurse said that her stomach really looks great. The thrush in her mouth is almost gone.

She'll be home soon. Our dreams will really be fulfilled. So many times it has seemed that our little girl would be taken from us, but God is a powerful Savior.

Empty Bed

February 6, 1976 — Friday

Barry and I went to see the baby today. She's still on the IVAC machine. The nurse said she cried a lot today.

She was sitting up asleep with blankets stacked behind her head.

I held her for a while. She woke up. When we had to leave, she was just wiggling her toes and looking all around.

Dr. Hamilton said he would be out of town all next week. He will have the resident doctor tell us when Natalie can go to the private room so I can learn to feed her through the tube.

Her color looks great. All the yellow is gone. The thrush is almost gone. The rash on her bottom looks good. Her stomach looks absolutely wonderful.

She'll be 12 weeks old this next week.

February 11, 1976 — Wednesday

Susan took mother and me to see Natalie today. She was awake when I got there — just looking all around. She really recognizes me. She just craves for me to touch and hold her close to me.

I held her for about 45 minutes. When I put her back in the bed, she cried till they propped her up.

She was sucking on her little fingers when I

left.

BARRY:

One of the nurses got something started while Natalie was in Intensive Care that would stick with her. She wasn't allowed a pacifier or anything, and because of the tube, wasn't given a bottle for sometime, so the nurse stuck her fingers in her mouth. She kept herself content for hours with just those three little fingers.

Cathy's Diary
February 12, 1976 — Thursday

She is 13 weeks old. She weights six pounds, six ounces — the most she's ever weighed.

February 13, 1976 — Friday

Michele took me to see Natalie today. We stayed about 50 minutes. I held my baby for part of that. She just stares at me. I sat her up so she could wiggle some.

Something happens inside me when she smiles. We just had a great time looking at each other. I told her "I love you!" at least 30 times. She eats it up.

They are going to do more blood tests on her. There are so many holes in her fingers and toes and all over her whole body. They've run out of

Empty Bed

places for needles to go.

Plus, they've had to shave her head at least four or five times.

CATHY:

We hadn't bought a bed for Natalie yet. I mean, we kept confessing that she would be coming home soon, and yet we didn't have a bed for her.

Now, I know things like that probably don't bother anyone but it really got to me. My mother said, "You don't have to worry about it. You just think about Natalie."

But it did bother me, and I said, "By faith, we are going to get a bed." We did. We set it up right in front of our bed.

I guess visitors thought that we were a bit "touched" — I mean, our daughter was still in Intensive Care down in Charlotte, and we were concerned about a bed for her in our home.

But it was just that settled. To others, including the medical staff, Natalie was constantly on the brink of developing something to destroy the delicate balance of her life. To us, she was just days from coming home to be with her mama and daddy.

Cathy's Diary
February 15, 1976 — Sunday

Another problem! Barry and I went to see Natalie today. The doctor said she developed a little blister, like a sore, on her stomach wound. It came yesterday and popped the same day.

They've never seen one quite like it. They don't know where it came from. Said they don't know if they'll have to do another biopsy.

Doctor Hamilton will decide. They took a culture from the blister's fluid.

Her bowel movements are not too normal looking. Is something still wrong with her liver, or is it something else?

God said, "Lean on me." She is in his hands. He is protecting her like he promised through prophecy. He alone is powerful.

February 17, 1976 — Tuesday

They did a scan today — shot dye in her veins to show if her liver is working properly.

She has lost weight down to six pounds, one ounce.

February 19, 1976 — Thursday

Natalie is three months old today. It's painful to think back to that November 19th and all that has happened since then.

Empty Bed

Barry talked to Dr. Hamilton by phone today. The doctor said that the tests showed that her liver was secreting some bile, but not enough. They are going to try a new drug on her so it will help her liver.

The doctor also said if she would just gain weight and keeping taking food, it would eliminate a lot of the problems.

God says she is healed, and that's all I have to stand on. He never fails, even when it looks like it.

February 20, 1976 — Friday

Jeff took me to see Natalie. She gained one ounce. I talked to one of the doctors. He said that the lab test showed that Natalie was secreting some bile from the liver into the intestines. "Not that much," he said, "but there must be a small passage or opening for it to go through." Potentially dangerous.

February 22, 1976 — Sunday

Barry and I went to see our baby today. She is back up to six pounds, six ounces. Her bowel movements are like they should be again.

We held her for two hours. She felt Barry's face and smiled whenever we smiled at her. When I made a sad face, she made one too.

February 29, 1976 — Sunday

Barry and I went. Natalie weighs six pounds, 10 ounces. The most ever. Praise our wonderful father!

We put a little yellow diaper shirt on her. It's the first thing she has ever worn. It's just been diapers before. That's all.

This past week, the liver medicine made her constipated. It's always something. So they had to adjust everything again. With her stomach like it is, they certainly don't want to take chances with constipation.

March 5, 1976 — Friday

The bilirubin count and liver problem are gone. Praise God. It's official.

They took her off heart medicine today. She had a slight murmur, but we can't be swayed. God says she is healed.

She gained another ounce. Her stomach looks great. She is getting food both by the mouth and her IVAC.

We put a green diaper shirt on her and a bow in her hair. She smiles so pretty.

March 6, 1976 — Saturday

Barry and I went. She lost a little weight today. The nurse said that it was probably because she

Empty Bed

leaks milk out from her stomach tube.

We learned today that they x-rayed her heart after they took her off heart medicine — wanted to see if it had enlarged. It was normal. Praise our God!

March 9, 1976 — Tuesday

Mama and I went. It's a red letter day — another first for our baby.

The isolette was cut off so she can get used to room temperature. She's still in it, but this is the first time she's been exposed to room air all the time.

The doctors said they will put her in an open hospital bed soon whenever they get an approval from Dr. Hamilton.

March 11, 1976 — Thursday

Barry's mother and I went to see Natalie. She's gained one and one-half ounces.

Tomorrow — March 12th — I'm going to spend the entire day and night with my baby!

She will be put in a private room. I can get there at 9:30 in the morning. I have to do all the tending to her. If all goes well, she'll probably get to come home Saturday or Sunday.

Praise God. The excitement I feel inside is unreal! God is so great.

I got to give her a bath in a tub of water today. I

changed the dressing on her stomach tube. The nurses said I did it really well.

My life will be so complete with my baby home!

CATHY:

It was that Thursday that sticks out in my mind. They told me that I'd get to take her to her private room. I could hardly sleep all night.

For so long, they had kept telling Barry and me — "Maybe next month." Finally, I asked, "Barry, is she ever going to get to come home?"

But the day did come. I got to go in with her to a private room. I wasn't supposed to be there until later, but I could not restrain myself from going very early — eight or so.

When we got there, they took her to the room. I had little blankets and crocheted afghans which mother and Aunt Betty had made. I got to take all that in.

They had a couch in there that I could lay on. I stayed there a week.

It really scared me to be all alone with my daughter. I was scared I didn't know how to do the stomach tube properly. It could pop out anytime.

I did pretty good, though. The nurses would come in. I'd ask, "How's this?" and point to the dressing. They'd say, "That's good."

Because it was a pediatrics ward, and because

of the unusual circumstances, I didn't eat much that week. I'd order my meals in the room, but they wouldn't bring me anything. I didn't want to go to the cafeteria and leave my baby all alone.

But it was worth it. I was with my baby. The time was getting close when we'd get to go home.

I faced that time with mixed emotions. On the one hand, I knew that she had beaten all the odds. It was impossible that she had made it this far. Honestly, no one would have ever dreamed — in the human sense — that she would actually be going home, especially if they had seen her that day four months before.

But on the other hand, it was a little terrifying to think about having to care for her at home. Most parents get panicky bringing home a "normal" baby who has had no complications; it's a pretty awesome thing to care for a helpless little infant.

But to bring home a baby with a stomach tube and so much supposedly still wrong with her — I have to admit that it is scary. I must keep trusting God for wisdom.

March 16, 1976 — Tuesday

Praise God! Natalie came home today at noon. It's been a long, long road. Somehow I feel that it's just beginning.

BARRY:

It's no coincidence that some of the most bothersome problems came just before Natalie was released from the hospital.

Nearly everytime — right before actually seeing the healing or situation solved — Satan always comes in to sidetrack.

But that's only to trap a person into believing that God isn't telling the truth.

God is not a liar. He wants to meet our needs. But it takes some standing and waiting. He never fails. He just isn't confined to our puny, little, human timetables.

Perhaps the head physician of pediatrics said it best: "Mr. Beaver, we did all we knew to do, but, truthfully, we had little do with your daughter's *real* healing."

10

CRUEL TAPE... SHAKING HANDS

CATHY:

I stayed with Natalie in the hospital for a week. Barry visited as much as he could. I think reality was starting to settle in.

What an unforgettable moment! Barry was down getting the car. I rode down in the elevator. One of the doctors was with me. He said, "It has been so many days Natalie has been in here. This is the day you've dreamed about, Mrs. Beaver!"

I could hardly contain my tears, so I just repeated what he said — "This *is* the day!"

I carried her in my arms down the elevator, got in the car with Barry's help and started towards

Kannapolis. Barry and I just kept looking at each other, then at the baby. We had looked forward to this day for so long, but with it finally happening, we were almost speechless.

BARRY:

We had a photographer there when we got home. We had a lot of time to make up. We overdid it, sure! We took pictures with her pretty clothes on. We took pictures with them off. We took pictures of her little stomach, the tube, everything. We acted crazy, I guess, but it was a real celebration. The Lord had vindicated his word.

Against all the odds, our little Natalie had come home to live with Cathy and me. How could we feel anything less than joy and parental happiness?

Still, there were those mixed emotions.

CATHY:

It was exciting to have Natalie with us in that bed we had bought in faith. But it was also a bit frightening when we realized that we had to care for our baby. There were no more nurses around to dote over her or doctors to take charge in case something went wrong.

She still had the tube in her stomach. I had been taught how to dress and bathe her with it still in.

But it was so much to do. Right after she would take a few ounces in a bottle, I'd have to keep her very still and level so that the milk would digest right. The nurses had told me that the tube could come out very easily — that if it did, I should immediately rush her back to the hospital because all the milk could come out of the hole where the tube was.

Well, that really left me shaky. I prayed the entire first two weeks after she came home — "Please don't let the tube come out!"

If she vomited a lot, I was to lay her flat in the bed, unclamp the tube and connect another tube to it and hang it up high so the milk could go up in that second tube and eventually drain a little at a time into her stomach.

So we had that to face. Every two hours, one of us was up giving Natalie her bottle, all the while praying, "God, please don't let her start vomiting!" I kept saying, "God, I'm not going to have to do that. She is not going to vomit!" She didn't — not even one time — even though she had many times throughout her stay in Intensive Care.

BARRY:

I had to dress Natalie's stomach tube for a while before Cathy would actually do it. It really tore our hearts out because of the incredible pain our little daughter had to go through.

There was this adhesive stuff that went on the tube and Natalie's skin, then the sticky tape over it. It was like putting adhesive tape onto contact cement, or something. When it touched, it stuck. It was imperative that this tube not be pulled out.

So every morning, I'd have to pull this tape off, use a liquid to wipe away the old adhesive, cleanse the entire area and start the sticky tape process over. When I'd get done, I was a "basket case." And Cathy would be crying. She knew what to do, but couldn't get herself to do it at home for a while. I had to do it.

If I had not been able then to walk out of the house, away from the pain, and go get my mind on something else, I would have cracked up.

Sometimes I wonder how either Cathy or I kept from totally flipping out. I just know that the Lord gave us the promise that he wouldn't bring anything on us that is greater than we can bear.

I don't know how we did it — the dressings, the pressure. I didn't want to do it. Neither did Cathy as she had to when I left for work early.

Dealing with the tension was one thing, but having it mount up and extra being added on — that was the real problem.

Dealing with it on a day-to-day basis was hard enough, but the extra things which went wrong were especially so.

It was like, "God, I just got on this level where I can really handle what is going on." Then, we'd wake up one morning and Natalie has this stuff running out of the tube all over her. We are 30-odd miles from our doctor. We certainly didn't want to take her to some other doctor who didn't know what had been going on for the past five months.

We were just in total mercy to what we had been taught, depending a thousand percent on the Holy Spirit's guidance to give some common sense to remember what to do, to keep calm enough so we could dress the tube right the first time.

That was important, especially with Natalie's dressing. I didn't want to goof it up. It had to be right. To redo it again meant just that much more pain for our little baby. I mean, the pain that she was going through was incredible enough, so it just had to be right the first time.

CATHY:

And baths — they were real problems. It was really a two-person operation, so I'd call mother — "Please, you've just got to come over here. I'm giving Natalie a bath now. Can you help?" I was just always nervous that something would go wrong — that the tube would mess up, or something would come loose.

But Natalie did great. We were in constant

contact with the doctor and, in three weeks, we went back in to stay in a private room at the Charlotte Memorial Hospital again for a week. They had some more things to do to Natalie — particularly with the stomach tube — if she had progressed enough. She had.

"I can't believe this is Natalie!" The nurses and doctors just raved over her. "She's gained so much weight." "She looks so good — and her color!"

When we got settled, Dr. Hamilton came into our room and said, "Well, she's doing real well. I'm going to take the tube out."

"When?"

"Now!" And he reached down with his hand and quickly jerked the stomach tube out. I almost crumbled. A wave of emotions hit me. That was the thing I had worked so hard to keep from happening — the tube to come out — for so long, and in an instant, the unthinkable had happened. The doctor had plopped it out with practiced precision. Just like that! Strangely enough, Natalie didn't cry or scream at all.

Then the doctor put a piece of gauze and tape over the dime-sized hole where the tube had been for so long — "We're going to see if we don't have to (he paused, searching for the right words) . . . if we can just leave it like it is — totally alone — and not have to stitch it up. If we have to go back with the needle, it'll just be more pain for her."

I thought, "Great! This will be good. She won't have anything else done to her. The hole will heal. We won't have any more problems."

Well, later when I started to feed her, the milk ran out like a sieve, gushing all over her stomach, between her legs, all on the sheet. I ran down the hall to get the nurse to help me. It was awful.

They kept wanting her to heal naturally, but I was changing her clothing and sheets many times a day. It got bad.

Three days later, I finally said, "You've just got to do something. It won't quit leaking."

So they took her back into a little room across the hall. It wasn't a full-fledged operating room — but some kind of surgery unit — and stitched her up. They had to stitch up a lot on the inside, they said, and some on the outside.

She came back screaming. I kept walking the floor. Mother was there with me.

"Natalie's going to be in great pain because we couldn't give much of anything to dull it," the doctor said.

So, I walked and carried her all that night — she just wouldn't stop crying.

BARRY:

We wondered if the pain would ever end. Would there always be something just around the corner lurking to mess everything up again? But we knew that every step also brought progress. It was that way when the tube was taken out of her stomach. At least we didn't have to do all that adhesive-thing anymore. Praise God for that!

We got to take Natalie home again in a few days, but the doctor warned, "When you take her back to Kannapolis, don't go anywhere with her for a month. I mean, don't go where people are, because if she should get a virus or cold, it could end everything."

So we lived by the letter of his law. She didn't go anywhere much for that month, and longer.

It was almost funny (if it hadn't been so serious). Some young people from the church wanted to see our baby so bad, so we let them look in the living room window!

Anytime even close relatives came, we'd slap a surgical mask on them before they even got through the front door.

Finally we took her to church. Well, sort of. We drove up there when the service was letting out, and Cathy held Natalie up to the car window for everyone to see her. They had heard so much about her, and so many of our fellow-believers had played such important roles as they interceded in prayer with us. Everybody really understood.

When we finally did take her out, especially to church, we wouldn't let anybody but a few relatives hold her. We had to be careful with her. People would even try to poke at her stomach!

We kept her at the very back of the church. I guess we were really funny about everything, but we had too much to gain to "blow it" at that stage.

When we went anywhere with Natalie, it looked like an ambulance service. We had extra gauze and dressings and bandages — just in case something happened. We were definitely prepared. If Natalie ever had any problems, we would automatically go into action.

CATHY:

After a while, if we were feeding her somewhere and she had a problem, it was less and less scary. We got more at ease, more proficient in taking care of her. We didn't get as upset.

But the problems were far from over. We had been home after the second hospital stay for only a month, when Natalie suddenly started jerking like she was going into some kind of seizure or something. Barry grabbed her and held her. For some reason, I called Jeff (my brother) and Michele. Normally I would have called our doctor, but it caught us so off-guard. We hadn't seen anything like these seizures before.

BARRY:

When Jeff and Michele got there, I was

holding Natalie. That was the first time that fear really gripped Cathy and me.

Up to that point, we had been soaring in our faith — like our faith in God had pulled us through this incredible thing — that we had licked every problem. The devil had lost.

But then that terrible, awful jerking started. She was seven months old by then. For a fleeting moment Satan brought that original fear which had gripped me so snake-like and tight, so crushingly powerful, that night when Natalie had been born.

I was crying. Cathy was crying. We thought our baby was dying or something. I thought, "Lord, you didn't bring us all the way to this point for this, did you? Not now, Lord!"

Jeff rushed in, laid his hands on Natalie, and prayed. Immediately, she stopped jerking. She stopped crying. The convulsion was over.

We found out later that they had her on phenobarbital during her time in the hospital, a drug given to epileptics, but they had certainly never said anything to us about her having convulsions or something similar.

CATHY:

That same thing happened some time later. I was home with her. Barry was gone. All of a sudden, she started doing that again — the jerking. I began confessing, "She is not going to

Cruel Tape . . . Shaking Hands

have another seizure like before!"

I rushed her to the Concord Children's Clinic. The doctor asked me in depth what had happened. The more I talked, the more he thought she had gone through a seizure. He wanted to put her right in the hospital, but I wanted to wait — "I have to talk to Barry first about this."

BARRY:

They came home. I got home about the same time from work. Cathy told me what the doctor had said. I said, "There is no way that we are taking her down there and letting a doctor who doesn't even know anything about her strap a bunch of instruments on her. There's no reason to do all those tests on just an isolated incident like this. We've seen her come too far just to slap her back in the hospital. We won't do it!"

CATHY:

I called the doctor the next day and told him what Barry and I had decided. I guess he thought we were nuts. But we had prayed and felt a peace about what we were doing.

BARRY:

We just purposed in our hearts that we would stand firm on it. We felt that it was just another little thing that the devil was using to shake our faith.

And when we made that decision, I saw — with my spiritual eyes — Satan look at me, turn around, and walk away. He knew then that he couldn't conquer us once, praise God, and he wasn't about to bring it on us again.

From that moment on, we really reached a stability in refusing any kind of negatives about Natalie's health.

11

THIS FAR BY FAITH

BARRY:

The faith walk we learned through Natalie has continued through some awfully murky waters. Anyone who tries to make it out to be anything else is playing games.

There's been no lack of problems. One of the worst came when Natalie was about a year old. She began crying one night and would not stop. This went on for hours. She just would not stop wailing. We could tell that she was in agonizing pain, but couldn't tell from what.

Finally, after praying, we rushed her in desperation to Presbyterian Hospital in Charlotte. We had already talked with our doctor, and he met us there.

Without any hesitation, he took her straight on in and began the examination. He thought she had an obstruction blocking something in there.

When they said "obstruction," Cathy and I joined together praying.

CATHY:

Fear gripped me at first until I came to my senses (spiritually) and realized that Jesus would just have to take control. We both walked the floor praying as they took Natalie to the X-ray unit.

The X-ray showed absolutely no obstruction, as the doctor originally feared. Now, whether there was one before, and God dissolved it, or if there never was, only he knows.

But the doctor's final prognosis was that she had been constipated, perhaps. He said to give her laxatives every night if necessary, and he made it clear that he never, never wanted her to get that way again.

BARRY:

But whether there had been an obstruction, or whether she was constipated all the time, — God intervened. When we left the hospital, Natalie was perfectly calm. That calmness had come in just a matter of minutes.

The problem happened again later. Natalie began having stomach cramps. The doctors wanted to go back in and find out what the problem was.

The doctor told us that Natalie's organs were not arranged like other human beings — not in the exact places. That first morning, they had such an incredible mass to deal with, they just wanted to get everything back in, get it closed up as quickly as possible and eliminate the risk of infection. At that point, it had only been a stopgap operation at best — a technicality to try to save a little newborn infant's life. They tried to get everything back in an approximate position, but they didn't want to drag the operation out too long. There was the constant fear that the baby would go into shock.

So, as Natalie did survive, and as she grew older, when the stomach cramps hit her, the doctor wanted to go back in to make sure that there were no problems. Plus, he wanted to put a mesh (she had no muscle in her stomach like others) and graft it to her skin — it would provide a muscular-like protection for her organs and flatten her stomach out.

But the doctor hit us with "a ton of bricks" when he said, "We don't really know what we will find when we go in there. The organs could actually be stuck together. The organs could even be stuck to the skin. There could be adhesions and lesions everywhere. Her organs could even be all hooked together."

CATHY:

I looked at the doctor and asked, "Can she die from an operation like this?" I didn't want any medical jargon or statistics. I just wanted to know. He looked back at me and said, "We don't know for sure. There are real dangers, sure." That was all I needed to know.

BARRY:

We asked for a little while to think about it. During that time, as we began praying, God did a special work on Natalie. Her stomach cramps ceased. When we went back in to tell the doctor that we didn't want the surgery, his entire attitude had changed. I said, "We just believe that God had something to do with the improvement. We are putting her into his hands." The doctor even changed his mind about operating.

I guess the medical people had gotten used to Cathy and me by then. Maybe they thought we were just two crazy Pentecostals when they first came in contact with us, but no one can argue with what God did.

The faith walk we have known since Natalie's ordeal has been filled with incredible victories, and horrible pitfalls.

We couldn't help but wonder, as time progressed, if — when we added to our family — we could be starting another horrible ordeal all over again. I think that it's a natural thought for any parent — especially for ones who had gone through what we had.

CATHY:

I just knew deep inside that when I had another child, it would be a boy. I hoped for this so Natalie wouldn't have to compare with another girl and ask why everything happened to her like it did.

But not long after Natalie's ordeal ended, God spoke to me in a prophecy, saying, "Yea, I say, my daughter, that there has been much fear in your life and fear must leave by my power.

"I say unto thee, it shall be but a short time, Yea, I say unto thee, that I am going to bring forth a new child.

"Yea, this child shall have my anointing upon it.

"Yea, it shall be a peculiar child. I say unto thee, it shall come forth shortly, by my power, saith the Lord your God."

On October 18, 1979, we *did* have another little girl, Leslie Annette. She was perfectly healthy. No complications. And she has been exactly like the prophecy — anointed.

She has been the perfect little sister for

Natalie — looking up to her "big" sister, trying to do everything she does. They couldn't be a more perfect pair. There really was no need for my fears about Leslie — God had it all under control even before she was conceived.

BARRY:

And God has continually taken us step by step. One of the most recent conflicts was the diagnosis that Cathy had cancer. God miraculously healed her.

For both of us, we can always go back to a home base when our faith really was born — the same night of Natalie's birth.

Anytime we are faced with struggles — small or mountainous — I can go back to that spot in my mind and remember that time in the Charlotte Memorial Hospital when God solidified my mind about holding on and believing and staring into the face of death. It's like — from that moment on — God moved in to let me know who was in control of everything.

Everything — beginning with that point — was just a continuing education. It really started with Natalie.

CATHY:

But it doesn't take something like Natalie's birth to bring faith into the forefront. The Word of God tells us to live a holy, unblemished life. He says to spend time preparing to know the Spirit of God who dwells within us (if we've accepted him). Then, if we are in tune with him, we can respond to any situation. Then, when we speak forth the words of faith, we can see results. In Romans 12:3, Paul wrote, "God hath dealt to every man the measure of faith." It's not some impossible dream; in fact, "Without faith, it is impossible to please him; for he that cometh to God must believe that he is, and that he is a rewarder of them that diligently seek him" (Hebrews 11:6).

The problems that come are for a purpose, as Peter wrote, "That the trial of your faith, being much more precious than of gold that perisheth, though it be tried with fire, might be found unto praise and honour and glory at the appearing of Jesus Christ."

That kind of faith is what God wants in each of us — a tried, unwavering faith like James described: "Let him ask in faith, nothing wavering. For he that wavereth is like a wave of the sea driven with the wind and tossed. For let not that man think that he shall receive any thing of the Lord."

That kind of tried, unwavering faith is the simple, pure kind — "What things soever ye desire, when ye pray, believe that ye receive them, and ye shall have them" (Mark 11:24).

God's promises are believed by the heart, but

the faith-filled believer also knows that his mouth must make the confession — "In the name of Jesus!"

For me, like Barry, the real understanding of faith began that dark night Natalie was born. Like Barry, it's the home base I go back to.

> *Don't be discouraged with trouble*
> *in your life;*
> *He'll bear your burdens*
> *And move all discord and strife.*
>
> *Just remember the good things*
> *He has done;*
> *Things that seemed impossible,*
> *Oh! Praise Him for the vic-t'ries*
> *He has won.*
>
> *Oh, we've come this far by faith,*
> *Leaning on the Lord;*
> *Trusting in His holy Word.*
> *He's never failed us yet.*
> *Oh! We can't turn back,*
> *We've come this far by faith.*

12

SHARING THE LIGHT

BARRY:

God is the author of life. I don't know if King David knew as much as we do today when he wrote, "I will praise thee; for I am fearfully and wonderfully made" (Psalm 139:14a).

I learned enough from my college biology and anatomy classes to keep me in awe — that the average adult has 60 thousand billion cells, each with the same genetic blueprint, yet ultimately specialized for its own particular task. A human's heart pumps 2,000 gallons of blood each day through 60,000 miles of blood vessels — not only feeding the body, but also processing out waste. The eye, the hand, the foot... No one, not even today's builders of facsimile robot technicians, knows exactly how much the human body is worth.

It only stands to reason that if God designed and created such an incredible place for the soul to dwell, he is vitally interested in what happens to that body.

John wrote, "Beloved, I wish above all things that thou mayest prosper and be in health, even as thy soul prospereth" (III, 2).

And if God is that concerned about his children, it also stands to reason that he has a purpose in having each child prosper and be in health for a purpose.

CATHY:

I asked God why all of it happened — why Natalie was born like that, why we had to go through everything. At first, I was afraid to ask, but after some time I couldn't keep the question back. I really wanted to know *why*. "Why, God? There must be an answer." I guess I still didn't understand why, after living for the Lord all my life, it had happened to me.

It was sometime later, maybe two years after Natalie was born, I was in a television rally — Barry and I sang, then sat down. But Jeff (my brother) called everyone up front. We were praying, seeking God.

Then Jeff touched my head and began giving a

Sharing The Light

word specifically for me: "I have spared your household for a testimony of my power. Now you have this light, now share this light with others. And my daughter, you will go through another test, and you shall lean on me."

I knew then — he had spared Natalie to be a light to the world.

That prophecy was given just as I was in the initial stages of cancer, but God was faithful. He had begun a good work in our family.

That work has continued. By the time Natalie was four, she was singing in public. Leslie followed quickly in her older sister's footsteps. They were both saved and baptized in the Holy Spirit at a young age.

They've both been special, anointed children. From the first church services where they sang, people have noticed. Even though Barry and I sang also and shared Natalie's miracle birth, we have been blessed along with the other listeners.

And Natalie's light continues shining. People across the nation have since heard her sing; television audiences have heard Barry and me share. Somehow, though we are still in awe, we know that it's just the beginning.

BARRY:

It's hard to believe — when we see our little Natalie out there singing her heart out — that this is the same pitiful newborn baby who fell into a plastic bag held by Dr. Monroe at the Cabarrus Memorial Hospital so long ago, that she's the same infant who had a floating umbilical cord ("It wasn't connected!" the doctor kept saying), that she's the daughter who caused so much commotion from the first moment she arrived at Charlotte's Memorial Hospital, that she's the same bundle over whom the surgeons worked feverishly to stuff her organs back in and stretch the skin over to protect her fragile little stomach.

But there she is — singing, causing tears and touching hearts.

It's hard to believe, but it *shouldn't be*. Not after all we've seen. Not after all God has done. Not after all he's promised.

To God be the glory,
To God be the glory,
To God be the glory,
   For the things He has done.

MORE FAITH–BUILDING BOOKS FROM HUNTINGTON HOUSE

A Reasonable Reason to Wait, by Jacob Aranza, is a frank, definitive discussion on premarital sex — from the biblical viewpoint. God speaks specifically about premarital sex, according to the author. The Bible also provides a healing message for those who have already been sexually involved before marriage. This book is must reading for every young person — and also for parents — who really want to know the biblical truth on this important subject.

America Betrayed! by Marlin Maddoux. This hard-hitting book exposes the forces in our country which seek to destroy the family, the schools and our values. This book details exactly how the news media manipulates your mind. Marlin Maddoux is the host of the popular, national radio talk show "Point of View."

Backward Masking Unmasked, by Jacob Aranza. Rock 'n' roll music affects tens of millions of young people and adults in America and around the world. This music is laced with lyrics exalting drugs, the occult, immorality, homosexuality, violence and rebellion. But there is a more sinister danger in this music according to the author. It's called "backward masking." Numerous rock groups employ this mind-influencing technique in their recordings. Teenagers by the millions — who spend hours each day listening to rock music — aren't even aware the messages are there. The author clearly exposes these dangers.

Backward Masking Unmasked, (cassette tape), by Jacob Aranza. Hear actual satanic messages and judge for yourself.

Close Calls, by Don Garlits, is the story of the thrills, triumphs and tragedies of a legendary American champion, "Big Daddy" Don Garlits. It is the heart-warming story of drag racing's most famous and popular driver. This book chronicles the many times "Big Daddy" has escaped death — both on and off the drag racing track. It is also a wonderful story of God's grace in his life.

Globalism: America's Demise, by William Bowen Jr. The Globalists — some of the most powerful people on earth — have plans to totally eliminate God, the family, and the United States as we know it today. Globalism is the vehicle the humanists are using to implement their secular humanistic philosophy to bring about their one-world government. The four goals of Globalism are *A ONE–WORLD GOVERNMENT * A NEW WORLD RELIGION * A NEW ECONOMIC SYSTEM * A NEW RACE OF PEOPLE FOR THE NEW WORLD ORDER. This book clearly alerts Christians to what the Globalists have planned for them.

God's Timetable for the 1980's, by Dr. David Webber. This book presents the end-time scenario as revealed in God's Word. It deals with a wide spectrum of subjects including the dangers of the New Age Movement, end-time weather changes, outer space, robots and biocomputers in prophecy. According to the author, the mysterious number 666 is occurring more and more frequently in world communications, banking and business. This number will one day polarize the computer code marks and identification numbering systems of the Antichrist, he says.

Murdered Heiress... Living Witness, by Dr. Petti Wagner.

The victim of a sinister kidnapping and murder plot, the Lord miraculously gave her life back to her. Dr. Wagner — heiress to a large fortune — was kidnapped, tortured, beaten, electrocuted and died. A doctor signed her death certificate, yet she lives today!

Praise Every Day, by Muriel Larson. This is a devotional guide which encourages the reader to center on praise during times of prayer. This exceptional book is particularly appropriate as a gift.

Rest From the Quest, by Elissa Lindsey McClain. This is the candid account of a former New Ager who spent the first 29 years of her life in the New Age Movement, the occult and Eastern mysticism. This is an incredible inside look at what really goes on in the New Age Movement.

Take Him to the Streets, by Jonathan Gainsbrugh. Well-known author David Wilkerson says this book is "... immensely helpful..." and "... should be read..." by all Christians who yearn to win lost people to Christ, particularly through street ministry. Effective ministry techniques are detailed in this how-to book on street preaching. Carefully read and applied, this book will help you reach other people as you *Take Him to the Streets*.

The Agony of Deception, by Ron Rigsbee. This is the story of a young man who became a woman through surgery and now, through the grace of God, is a man again. Share this heartwarming story of a young man as he struggles through the deception of an altered lifestyle only to find hope and deliverance in the grace of God.

The Day They Padlocked the Church, by Ed Rowe. This is the warm yet heartbreaking story of Pastor Everett Sileven, a Nebraska Baptist pastor, who was jailed and his church padlocked because he refused to bow to Caesar. It is also the story of 1,000 Christians who stood with Pastor Sileven in defying Nebraska tyranny in America's crisis of freedom.

The Divine Connection, by Dr. Donald Whitaker. This is a Christian guide of life extension. It specifies biblical principles on how to feel better and live longer. Dr. Whitaker says you really *can* feel better and live longer and shows you how to experience Divine health, a happier life, relief from stress, a better appearance, a healthier outlook on life, a zest for living and a sound emotional life.

The Hidden Dangers of the Rainbow, by Constance Cumbey. A national #1 bestseller, this is a vivid expose' of the New Age Movement which is dedicated to wiping out Christianity and establishing a one-world order. This movement — a vast network of tens of thousands of occultic and other organizations — meets the test of prophecy concerning the Antichrist.

The Hidden Dangers of the Rainbow Tape, by Constance Cumbey. Mrs. Cumbey, a trial lawyer from Detroit, Michigan, gives inside information on the New Age Movement in this teaching tape.

Training for Triumph, by Dr. George Selig. Here is a parents' manual to help you learn good techniques on successful parenting and child raising. Dr. Selig, Professor of Special Education at CBN University, Virginia Beach, Virginia, explains how to apply proven biblical principles and teachings while children are still young.

The Twisted Cross, by Joseph Carr. One of the most important works of our decade, *The Twisted Cross* clearly documents the occult and demonic influence on Adolf

Hitler and the Third Reich which led to the Holocaust killing of more than six million Jews. The author even gives the specifics of the bizarre way in which Hitler actually became demon-possessed.

Who Will Rise Up? by Jed Smock. This is the incredible — and sometimes hilarious — story of Jed Smock, who, with his wife Cindy, has preached the uncompromising gospel on the malls and lawns of hundreds of university campuses throughout this land. They have been mocked, rocked, stoned, mobbed, beaten, jailed, cursed and ridiculed by the students. Yet this former university professor and his wife have seen the miracle-working power of God transform thousands of lives on university campuses.

Yes, send me the following books and/or tapes:

___ copy (copies) of **A Reasonable Reason To Wait** @ $4.95 = ___
___ copy (copies) of **America Betrayed!** @ $5.95 = ___
___ copy (copies) of **Backward Masking Unmasked** @ $4.95 = ___
___ copy (copies) of **Backward Masking Unmasked Cassette Tape** @ $5.95 = ___
___ copy (copies) of **Close Calls** @ $6.95 = ___
___ copy (copies) of **Globalism: America's Demise** @ $6.95 = ___
___ copy (copies) of **God's Timetable For the 1980's** @ $5.95 = ___
___ copy (copies) of **Murdered Heiress ... Living Witness** @ $5.95 = ___
___ copy (copies) of **Praise Every Day** @ $10.95 = ___
___ copy (copies) of **Rest From the Quest** @ $5.95 = ___
___ copy (copies) of **Take Him to the Streets** @ $6.95 = ___
___ copy (copies) of **The Agony Of Deception** @ $6.95 = ___
___ copy (copies) of **The Day They Padlocked the Church** @ $3.50 = ___
___ copy (copies) of **The Divine Connection** @ $4.95 = ___
___ copy (copies) of **The Hidden Dangers of the Rainbow** @ $4.95 = ___
___ copy (copies) of **The Hidden Dangers of the Rainbow Seminar Tapes** @ $13.50 = ___
___ copy (copies) of **Training for Triumph** @ $4.95 = ___
___ copy (copies) of **The Twisted Cross** @ $7.95 = ___
___ copy (copies) of **Who Will Rise Up?** @ $5.95 = ___

AT BOOKSTORES EVERYWHERE or order direct from: Huntington House, Inc, P.O. Box 53788, Lafayette, LA 70505.

Send check/money order or for faster service VISA/Mastercard orders call toll-free 1-800-572-8213. Add: Freight and handling, $1.00 for the first book ordered, 50¢ for each additional book.

Enclosed is $ _____ including postage.

Name _____

Address _____

City _____ State and Zip _____